BEYOND STRETCHING:
RUSSIAN FLEXIBILITY BREAKTHROUGHS

**BY PAVEL TSATSOULINE,
MASTER OF SPORTS**

Dragon Door Publications, Inc.
St. Paul, Minnesota

Published in the United States by:

Dragon Door Publication, Inc
PO Box 4381, St. Paul, MN 55104

Tel: (651) 645-0517
Fax: (651) 644-5676

E-mail: dragondoor@aol.com

Website: www.dragondoor.com

ISBN: 0-938045-18-0

Produced by Patrick D. Gross
Book Design by Jennifer Closner
Digital photography by Scott Jacobson
Digital photography for Second Edition by Andrea Du Cane
Photographs from *Beyond Stretching* video, courtesy Precision Tapes, Inc

Manufactured in the United States

First Edition: May 1997
Second Edition: November 1998

DISCLAIMER

The author and publisher of this material are not responsible in any manner whatsoever for any injury which may occur through following the instructions contained in this material. The activities, physical and otherwise, described herein for informational purposes only, may be too strenuous or dangerous for some people and the reader(s) should consult a physician before engaging in them.

To Julie

I have trained Soviet commandos to
DO SPLITS IN THREE
TO SIX MONTHS—
whether they liked it or not.
Soviet Spetsnaz,
the Special Operations Forces,
were combat ready 24 hours a day
and did not have the luxury of a
warmup and stretch before going
into action. I have trained my men to
DISPLAY MAXIMAL
FLEXIBILITY COLD.
Now that I have turned into a
capitalist running dog, I will teach you too.
When I'm done with you, you'll have
the flexibility of a mutant.
Or else.

Pavel Tsatsouline,
Master of Sports

CONTENTS

PART ONE: NERD STUFF

Part One: Nerd Stuff

Twilight of the flexibility idols

Most Western flexibility "experts" do not know enough physiology to have sex. You are far better off not stretching at all than following their advice:

The more flexible one is, the better. You can't be too flexible.

Flexibility improves performance in any sport.

Flexibility is the key to injury prevention.

You will get injured if you don't warm up and stretch before exercise.

Injuries occur when a muscle is stretched beyond its limit.

A stretch must be slow and steady. Dynamic stretching is dangerous and counterproductive.

You must stretch every day.

It takes years to achieve reasonable flexibility and it is lost quickly.

You will never be able to do splits unless you started very young.

Very few males have the potential to do splits.

You have to elongate your muscles, tendons and ligaments in order to become more flexible.

Every one of these flexibility commandments is wrong. The fact that everybody repeats them like the Communist party line does not change it.

Never assume the obvious is true.

Why the American approach to flexibility failed

Hackers have a saying, "Garbage in, garbage out." If the premise is false, the conclusions will be wrong.

The American approach to flexibility has failed because it starts with the assumption that muscles and connective tissues need to be physically stretched. Other myths snowball from there.

Your muscles have plenty of length to allow you to do splits, for instance. As long as you have healthy joints, it is only your own tension that is preventing you from going all the way down.

Having a hard time buying it? Try this test. Can you extend one leg to the side at a 90 degree angle?

Your leg that is up on the table is now in the position for a side split.

Now, listen to this: no muscles run from one leg to the other. That means you should be able to bring the other leg out at the same angle and do a split without stretching a thing.

So why can't you?

Your body feels funny about having your legs at an angle they have never been at before. You have to reeducate your nervous system into believing that it's safe. Only then will it allow your muscles to relax into the new position. *Beyond Stretching* will teach you how to develop extreme flexibility by tricking the muscle into relaxing and picking up the slack.

★

I bet my autopsy reveals my mouth is too big.

Calvin,
Tiger Hobbes' buddy

★

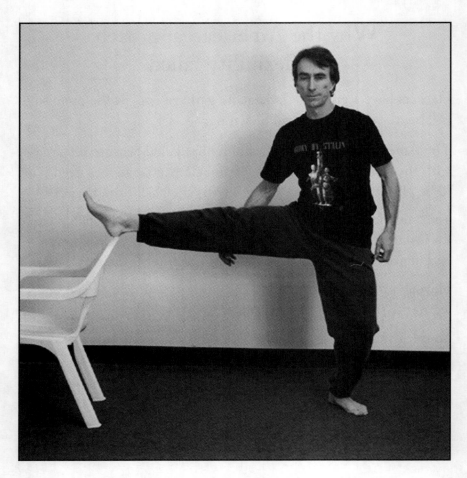

If you can do this, nothing stops you from doing the splits.

Aging and flexibility:
what can and can't be done

What if your age qualifies you for Social Security? It will still work.

Americans lose flexibility as they grow older because they are used to relying on the elasticity of their tissues.

A lifetime of activity causes micro trauma in our muscles. When a muscle heals, scar tissue is formed. The scar tissue pulls the wound together making the muscle shorter. American doctors believe that relaxed stretching after exercise can prevent the muscle from healing at a shorter length.

I know an aerobic instructor who developed a barbaric stretching method based on this theory. She purposefully tears her hamstrings by over stretching them, then spends hours in that position to insure that the muscles will heal at a new, increased, length. High quality S&M material, if you are into that sort of thing.

Even if you can prevent the muscle from shortening—and that is questionable—a stiffening of the connective tissues is as sure as death and taxes. Soviet scientist and physician Alexander Bogomoletz said "Man is as old as his connective tissues."

Ligaments and tendons are made of *collagen* which gives them strength, and *elastin*, which, as its name implies, provides elasticity. With time the elastic/collagen ratio changes in favor of collagen, or scar tissue. The process is irreversible. Slowing it down by being active—and it doesn't have to be stretching—is the best you can hope for.

Bottom line. If you rely on tissue elasticity for flexibility, you will lose it.

★

There isn't an exercise that can prevent aging of connective tissues. It's as certain as radioactive isotope decay.

—Academician Nikolay Amosov, USSR

★

Stretching is NOT the solution to remaining flexible. Trying to change the mechanical properties of your muscles, tendons and ligaments is a desperate way to become flexible and works well only in children.

Fortunately, a muscle with pre-Depression connective tissues and more scars than a prize fighter, is still long enough to display as much flexibility as allowed by its associated joints.

Master the regulation of muscular tension, and you will be as flexible as you want to be—at any age.

Flexibility and "damage control" in low-grade injuries

Do you feel like a kid who just learned that there is no Santa Claus? Too bad. Here goes the Tooth Fairy:

> *"Injuries occur when a muscle is stretched beyond its limit.*
> *So prevent injuries by elongating the muscles and*
> *connective tissues."*

Wrong on both accounts. According to Eastern Bloc research, a muscle does not have to be maximally stretched to be torn. Muscle tears are the result of a special combination of a sudden stretch and a contraction.

Say, you slip on ice. Your body is thrown off balance. It will reflexively try to recover. The muscle that was stretched when you slipped, probably groin or hamstring, will contract to return to the position it was in. Here we have it. A stretch from one side, a contraction from the other. The tissue tears.

This involuntary contraction is called the *stretch reflex*. A muscle that is stretched by an external force too far or too fast will contract to oppose the stretch.

Can anything be done to prevent this?

"Prevent" is a strong word—ask your lawyer. "Improve the odds" is more accurate. You already know that "elongating" the tissues is a dumb idea. Instead, reset the sensitivity of the stretch reflex so it will not fire too soon. This is done by gradually increasing the range and speed of your stretches.

Why flexibility is speed specific— the case for *dynamic flexibility stretching*

Yes, "speed!" Another flexibility myth is about to bite the dust— the one that prescribes stretching slow and steady and warns against bouncing.

Remember, the stretch reflex clicks in when the muscle is stretched either too far or too fast. There are two types of receptors, or *muscle spindles*, that trigger the stretch reflex. One receptor is sensitive to the magnitude of the stretch. The other receptor is sensitive to the magnitude and speed of the stretch. Static stretching will reset the former receptor, but not the latter.

So flexibility is speed specific.

To be flexible in motion, you have to stretch in motion— eventually at the velocity of your sport.

This is a complete turnaround from the wide spread paranoia about the supposed dangers of fast movement. Ironically, some tissues are less prone to an injury when they are stressed rapidly.

The ligaments are partly made up of wavy collagen fibers. If you uncoil them, the fibers become taut and injury prone. Stretched six to eight percent above its resting length, a ligament tears.

Slow loading picks up the protective slack in the "coils," while a quickly applied force usually does not have enough time to do it.

★

"If the meek ever inherit the earth, our defensive line is going to wind up owning Texas."

—Jerry More, football coach

★

11

Studies show that knee ligaments withstand fifty percent more force when the speed of loading is increased!

Joint surfaces are also much less likely to get damaged when loaded fast because of certain properties of the cartilage.

Cartilage is the tissue sandwiched between the joint surfaces. It decreases the joint stress by reducing friction and distributing the load over a large area of the joints.

Cartilage is twenty to forty percent collagen and sixty to eighty percent water. Predictably, it acts like a water soaked sponge when compressed. The fluid is squeezed out, thinning the protective padding between the bones.

When the loading is rapid, as in landing from a jump, the water does not have enough time to get squeezed out, and cartilage shock absorbing qualities are at their highest.

Bottom line. Human bodies were not built for "Nautilus." Ballistic movement is the natural way for us to operate.

Does this mean that dynamic flexibility training is 100% safe?

No, it doesn't. But neither is conventional relaxed stretching.

Dr. James Garrick, medical advisor to the NFL, U.S. Figure Skating Team, and the San Francisco Ballet, has pointed out that this kind of stretching is one of the fastest growing causes of injuries in the US.

By subjecting yourself to the minor risk of an occasional muscle pull when you stretch in motion, you will considerably improve your odds against a more serious injury when you practice your sport or slip on a banana peel. The stretch reflex won't fire and you won't pull anything. And if you want to play it really safe, stick to Trivial Pursuit.

Do you really need to warmup? Or, what happened to the emperor's clothes?

"You will get injured if you don't warm up and stretch before exercise."

I'm going to burst your bubble. There is no scientific evidence that a conventional warmup and/or stretching before you do something active decreases the possibility of an injury or improves your performance.

Silly experiments are conducted to "prove" the "need" for warmups. In a recent one evil geeks ripped a rabbit's muscle at 37 degrees Celsius, its normal temperature, then at 40 degrees. Apparently, it took more force to tear the thing at a higher temp. A frozen rubber band snaps easier than a warm one, you've heard the analogy before.

Fortunately for the rabbits, they haven't. The species would have been long extinct. "Excuse me, Mr. Big Bad Wolf, I need to ride my stationary bike and do some quad stretches before I run for my life."

Surprise: according to Soviet research, in wild animals and properly conditioned people the physiological changes needed for fight or flight—such as increased temperature, fluid viscosity, circulation and muscle tone—take only seconds to develop. It is a necessity of survival and you do not learn these things in the safety of your lab.

I come from a world where they eat their young and evolution is still at work. My advice is more practical. If you cannot perform at full throttle when the shit hits the fan—you are lunch.

★

"Some ideas are so stupid, only intellectuals believe them."

—H.G. Wells

★

13

Beyond warmups: developing round-the-clock readiness for action

Save your pet story about getting injured when you did not warm up. Too bad for you. If you always warm up and stretch before exercise, your body starts expecting it and will not perform well without it. Hence, the injury. It is also in your head. Research suggests that warmup benefits only those who believe they need it. And even that is not always the case.

Dr. Judd Biasiotto, one of the smartest guys to wear sneakers since Einstein, and I'm not kidding, did a study on the baseball practice of warming up with a lead bat. It was believed to increase the bat velocity. The question the owners of the Kansas City Royals were asking was not whether the batting speed increased, but rather by how much.

He found that FORTY-SEVEN OUT OF FIFTY PROFESSIONAL BASEBALL PLAYERS TESTED HAD A BETTER BAT VELOCITY WITHOUT A WARMUP. Curiously, they all believed it was the other way around. Since the difference in speed was minor, the team management decided to stick with the tradition, so the vulnerable psyches of the players would not be traumatized.

So stop being a head case! Gradually wean yourself off warmups and eventually drop them entirely.

You can improve your readiness for action much more effectively with dynamic flexibility training. No, I am not contradicting myself. You will be through with these drills long before the wolf shows up. Read on.

Dynamic stretches allow you to reset your nervous regulation of muscular length and tension, on both a short and long term basis.

★

"The body becomes its function."

—Bulgarian athletes' credo

★

14

They enable you to display your current maximal flexibility without a warmup for the rest of the day, no matter how out of shape you are.

In Spetsnaz we were required to do high kicks before breakfast. As a result we could do them later in the day whenever the situation called for it. Eventually, we could kick even if we did not get to stretch in the morning. That's the long term effect. A wild thing at last.

Beyond dynamic stretching:
Plyometric Flexibility Training

Most athletes should do dynamic/plyometric stretching before a competition. This way you can be 100 percent ready the moment you begin. Why yield even a second's advantage to your opponent?

If you ever watched international track-and-field meets, you may have noticed that while western athletes waste their time with slow static stretches, the Russians and East Germans are bouncing around. They aren't just stretching. The benefits of this *Plyometric Flexibility Training* go beyond flexibility. Jumping around speeds up the heart rate which in turn stimulates the adrenal response. The neural input to your muscles is also increased and the stretch reflex is "sharpened."

It "sharpens" your stretch reflex and increases the neural input to your muscles.

There is more to the stretch reflex than its contribution to muscle injuries. The reflex is what puts a "spring" into your movement. A muscle that has been sharply stretched generates much more force than a static muscle. Try pitching a baseball without a windup and you will know what I am talking about.

There are two reasons for that. First, a larger number of motor units are recruited reflexively than voluntarily. And second, like a rubber band, your muscles and tendons are elastic and tend to return to their resting length after they have been stretched.

To ensure that extra boost, the transition from stretch to shortening, or loading, must be quick, otherwise the stored elastic energy dissipates as heat. This quickness is referred to as the *reactive ability*. It is developed with *plyometrics*—a Russian discovery, naturally.

Plyometrics are various jumps and other exercises that condition you to make the quickest "touch-and-go." Ballistic flexibility drills are a form of plyometrics.

Now you see why your Mom and apple pie relaxed stretching does not help—just the other way around. It "flattens" your stretch reflex and compromises your explosiveness. Besides, like a rubber band, tissues stretched beyond their point of restitution remain permanently over stretched and lose some of their elasticity.

A rag doll cannot act like a spring.

Plyometrics, on the other hand, improve your tissues' viscoelasticity.

Another benefit of plyometrics in general, and plyometric stretching specifically, is the increased neural input to the muscles.

Your nervous system is very efficient and recruits only as much muscle as it takes to get the job done. Strangely, a given level of neurological activity will be maintained for some time after the demand has been imposed. The involuntary raising of your arms after you push against the doorway is an example of this phenomenon.

Remember that a reflexive muscular contraction utilizes more motor units than a voluntary one. For a short time after the stretch reflex has been employed your body maintains the ability to contract the target muscle harder than usual, even at will.

Thanks to the phenomenon of *residual recruitment*, plyometrics, unlike the traditional warmup and stretching, DOES improve your immediate performance in speed-strength sports such as sprint, high jump, or powerlifting.

Alternatives to warm up in weight training— why the *ramp* is better than the *pyramid*

Bulgarian weight lifters don't warm up or stretch before lifting a maximal weight, and they are the best in the world, along with Russians.

If you train yourself to excel at something, you should be able to do it when the KGB drags you out of bed at four A.M.

Most American lifters warm up using the "pyramid" concept. They start their workouts with a light weight and increase it every set while decreasing the reps. Once the max is achieved, the sequence is reversed. An example would be: 12, 10, 8, 6, 4, 2, 1, 2, 4, 6, 8, 10, 12 repetitions. Each set is taken to, or close to, failure.

The last time the Soviets used this cutting edge technique was 1964.

It comes as a surprise to most Americans who train with weights that strength training is not about exhausting the muscles quickly— that's bodybuilding. Strength training requires maintaining a high force output for as long as possible without fatigue. The pyramid caused premature fatigue and had to go.

★

"Lower skilled people…use the first rep as a body awareness tool. As they become more skilled, their first rep will be their best."

—Louie Simmons, powerlifting coach extraordinaire

★

You may argue that, even if warming up the muscles is not important or perhaps counterproductive, the pyramid allows a lifter to get into the groove of an exercise with a light weight before nailing the heavy sets.

In case of a beginner, or with a new exercise, the point is well taken. However a technique called "ramping" allows you to achieve the same effect without the unnecessary fatigue. As opposed to pyramiding, you ramp up with low reps and go nowhere near muscle failure. Here is an example of how two athletes work up to a 400 pound squat using the pyramid and the ramp:

Pyramid	Ramp
135 x 20	135 x 5
225 x 12	225 x 3
315 x 8	315 x 1
365 x 6	365 x 1
385 x 3	405 x 1
405 x 1	

Ramp by what feels right, or use this standard progression:

> 50% x 3
> 70% x 2
> 90% x 1
> 100–120% x 5–10 seconds hold * (optional)
> 100% x 1, or whatever repetitions your top set calls for

* For example, holding the weight in a locked out position for the bench press, or standing with a barbell on your shoulders for squatting. Supporting a supramaximal weight before lifting a maximal weight will make your max feel a lot lighter by comparison. Try it, it works! If you want to know why and would like to learn about the latest breakthroughs in strength training, check out *The Rocket Science of Strength Training*, a soon-to-be-released book I have coauthored with Dr. Fred Clary.

An accomplished lifter does not need either form of preparation, with a possible exception of a short ramp for the dead lift and new exercises.

The few people in the States who train without a warmup are simply too stupid to understand its "importance." Four times powerlifting world record holder Judd Biasiotto, Ph.D is an exception.

"Biasiotto… remained fast asleep," wrote a lifter who witnessed Dr. Judd's unorthodox performance. "When but five lifters had yet to lift, Biasiotto's coach woke him.

Judd rose, pulled up the straps of his suit, and started wrapping his knees. I had to laugh. How could such a strong athlete be so foolish as to miss his warmups?

"Just another powerlifting moron," I thought. "That's all this clown is."

But when Biasiotto stepped on the platform to attempt his opening lift, my opinion changed drastically. Within less than ten seconds, he brought about a physiological transformation that could only be described as bizarre. His facial features seemed to change before my eyes. The hair on his arms and legs stood up, and his breathing became deep and rhythmic. His muscles actually seemed to increase in size. The whole scene was a little scary.

Without a single warmup, Biasiotto unracked the weight, descended, and then exploded up with it for a new Georgia State record. The lift was ridiculously easy.

Eight more times during the meet, Biasiotto repeated his astonishing transformation, and eight more times he made seemingly effortless lifts. By the end of the day, Biasiotto had surpassed ten state records and captured the outstanding lifter's award."

"Dr. Judd," as he is known to the powerlifting community, conducted a study involving other advanced powerlifters to prove he was not a freak of nature. One group warmed up before performing maximum lifts, the other didn't. Now, eat this. FIVE OUT OF SIX TIMES THE NON-WARMUP GROUP SHOWED BETTER RESULTS in the squat and the bench press! Dr. Judd explained it as the "absence of warmup induced fatigue."

The deadlift was a different story. In all six studies the warmed up subjects did better. Dr. Biasiotto speculated that the deadlift is a "mind lift." The "dead" weight just sits there looking impossible to move. You do not get a chance to feel the weight and judge how much force is needed to lift it and whether it is within your abilities.

The control group lifters must have got psyched out without the reassurance of gradually increasing lifts. All of them expressed fear and anxiety before the deadlift. There was none of that before the other two powerlifts, because, Dr. Judd surmised, in the squat and bench press you get the feel for the weight when you lower it.

By the way, there were no injuries in the study, although over 500 of maximal or near maximal lifts were made. If beginning lifters were studied, the results might have been different, both in performance and injury rate. Untrained bodies take longer to get primed for action. Too long to survive one bad Saturday night in Moscow.

★

"I don't care how flexible you are. I'll tie your ankles to two jeeps, floor 'em— and you are history."

—A Soviet
Special Ops DI

★

Extreme range strength: the key to damage control in high-force accidents

Russians knew for a long time that flexibility alone is helpful only in reducing minor soft tissue injuries. The stretch reflex doesn't fire and you don't pull anything. It is a different ball game if the force acting upon you exceeds the structural integrity of your tissues.

Flexibility becomes a liability.

In an inflexible person the muscle reflexively contracts to absorb the force, often tearing in the process. It was meant to. Soft tissue is sacrificed to spare the slow healing tendons and ligaments. It is damage control.

A flexible person who has removed his or her first line of defense, the stretch reflex, will suffer a much more serious connective tissue injury. Here is what happened to a hyperflexible national level aerobics competitor:

The woman was water skiing and her foot got caught by the tow cable. Her hip was forcefully abducted, or pulled out to the side. The athlete's deconditioned stretch reflex did not turn on while it still could save the connective tissue at the price of a muscle tear. When it did, it was too late. The momentum was too great and the hip was in a vulnerable fully open position. What could have been a groin strain in an inflexible mere mortal, became a joint and ligament whiplash injury in the hyper-flexible aerobic junky. The young woman's leg was literally hanging on a few shreds of tissue when it was over. Fortunately, American orthopedic surgeons tend to do a better job than the stretching "experts."

But don't give up your stretching yet. If a reflexive contraction isn't there, train to produce one at will.

Strength in the extreme, most vulnerable, range of motion, will give you a fighting chance of pulling out of such a predicament. If the water skier's groin muscles were strong, she would have been able to contract them even without the help from the stretch reflex. Her muscles would still probably have been torn, but her leg would not have been twisted out like a fried chicken's.

The best methods for extreme range strength development: full-range weight training and *Isometric Flexibility Training*

The obvious way to develop *extreme range strength* is by lifting weights. The only requirement is range specificity.

You get stronger primarily in the range where you train. If you can do full 180 degree splits, the health club adductor/abductor, or inner/outer thigh, machine limited to 120 degrees is worthless.

If you can't come up with a weight lifting exercise that trains your muscles in the extreme range, do isometrics.

You are probably familiar with *Isometric Strength Training*. It was very popular in the sixties. You had to push against things that didn't budge, like walls. Your muscles contracted but no movement happened. You got stronger at the angles you trained. Isometric training went out of vogue because the aerobic establishment hollered that it had no cardiovascular value. So it does not. I can think of a lot of fine things which offer no aerobic benefits. It does not change the fact that isometrics remains an effective method of strength training.

To develop extreme range strength with isometrics, stretch as far as you can, then flex the stretched muscle. The exact protocol is described in the next chapter.

Isometric stretching helps damage control by improving extreme range strength. But it offers many other benefits.

One is dramatically increased flexibility. Isometric stretching is documented to be at least 267% more effective than conventional relaxed stretching. It accomplishes this in a number of ways.

Relaxed stretching develops flexibility without strength. This is unnatural.

Normally your body does not allow a range of motion it cannot control. A graphic illustration of this is a medical condition known as the "frozen shoulder." If after an injury you do not use your shoulder for a long time it will lose much of its range of motion. Under anesthesia, though, the surgeon can turn the shoulder through 360 degrees without trouble.

When the patient wakes up and his muscles start working, the shoulder freezes again. The nervous system knows that the muscles are not strong enough to control the full range of motion and will not let the shoulder's owner have it.

When you become stronger in the extreme range of motion, you send the message to your body that you will not be stuck in that position, because you now have the strength to recover from it. Your muscles will not undergo a reflexive contraction since your nervous system perceives the stretch as safe. Your flexibility increases.

Another way isometric stretching makes you more flexible is by manipulating the stretch reflex. You can trick it, or cancel it out. The first method is used by U.S. physical therapists. It is a spelling test nightmare: *proprioceptive neuromuscular facilitation,* or *PNF.*

PNF works by fooling your stretch reflex. Here you are, stretched out to what your body thinks is the limit. The muscle does not seem to be able to get any tenser. Yet you make it happen by flexing that muscle. When you relax the muscle afterwards, it does not feel as tight as before and you can eke out a little more stretch.

Extreme flexibility through correct breathing

The effectiveness of PNF can be dramatically increased through proper breathing. Take a lesson from chi-kung, tai chi, and yoga. Masters of these Oriental disciplines put heavy emphasis on breathing exercises which leads to remarkable mastery of the body and the mind.* Here is why.

Your nervous system is subdivided into voluntary which is in charge of things like lifting your arm or chewing a cheeseburger, and autonomic which quietly runs things which are none of your business, like your heart rate and digestion.

Breathing is the only function you can control both consciously and unconsciously because it is regulated by both branches of the nervous system through two sets of nerves. By controlling your breathing you can control some of your body's functions which were never meant to be controlled voluntarily, like your heart rate. Note how forcing yourself to "take a deep breath" when you freak out helps to calm you down. Because deep, relaxed breathing is incompatible with a stressed out mind, your body adjusts its physiology to your breathing!

★

"Breathing is the bridge between mind and body, the connection between consciousness and unconsciousness."

—Andrew Weil, Harvard M.D.

★

* Dragon Door Publications carries a fine selection of books on chi kung. Call (800) 899-5111 for a free catalogue.

While curling a dumbbell or climbing stairs are voluntary acts, residual muscle tension is an autonomic function. You cannot control it directly, but by breathing in a pattern characteristic of a given level of muscular tension or relaxation you can make it happen! Note how powerlifters instinctively hold their breath when they are lifting a heavy weight. They are using a breathing—or rather "no breathing"!—pattern most appropriate for generating maximum muscular tension. You can do the same for inducing a deep muscular relaxation with Pneumomuscular Flexibility Training. Learn how in Part II.

Enter the heavy artillery:
Shutdown Threshold Isometrics

A kickboxer who practiced standard PNF diligently for years came to me as the last resort. He was only three inches off the ground in the side split, yet never got any deeper. "Experts" told him it was not meant to be, he was not built for splits and too old. With shutdown threshold isometrics I put him in a full Chinese split in ten minutes, screams notwithstanding.

I did it with Shutdown Threshold Isometrics, a revolutionary Russian technique which drops even untrained middle aged males into full splits in half a year or less. If standard PNF, or even Pneumomuscular Flexibility Training, fails you, STI will come through! I would save it as a last resort though, because it is extremely painful and exhausting.

Shutdown threshold isometrics, or STI, does not bother to trick the stretch reflex. It just cancels it out with another reflex, the *Golgi organ reflex*.

The GTR is the last line of defense against injuries. It takes over where the stretch reflex leaves off. As the muscle is fighting an

★

"I feel your pain, my fellow Americans."

—President Bill Clinton

★

25

overwhelming force it gets very tense. The Golgi tendon organ located at the junction of the muscle and tendon registers the tension. As it exceeds a certain level, the *shutdown threshold*, the/ GTO recognizes that the struggle is hopeless and collapses the muscle to prevent it from ripping its tendons off their attachments.

This mechanism is known as the *feedback loop*. You have run across its work when you had your ass kicked in arm wrestling. One moment your biceps is super tense, the next it goes jello.

Shutdown threshold isometrics trigger the GTR to relax a muscle so you can then stretch it. Half-assed contractions practiced by US physical therapists are way too wimpy to trigger the GTR. The tension must be extremely high. You must put weight on the stretched muscles and contract them to the extreme. It is very painful—scream your heart out.

Now, stop mumbling "Is it safe, is it safe?" You sound like the dentist from *The Marathon Man*.

Like everything else, STI is not fool-proof. What matters is that the benefits by far outweigh the risks. You'll be much more resistant to an injury:

> *The isometrics will make you more flexible and stronger in the extreme range of motion.*

> *Repeated application of high force on your tendons will make them thicker and stronger.*

> *You will have a higher shutdown threshold and that translates into even more strength for damage control.*

How to build super strength with the *feedback loop*

STI builds strength in two ways:

You improve your muscle activation.

You raise your previous shutdown threshold.

The threshold point is set up very conservatively. Much more force is needed for the tissue to rupture, than is determined by the threshold point. Studies show that the maximal voluntary strength of the muscle represents only 30% of the tensile strength. That leave a great safety margin.

Have you heard about people performing amazing feats of strength in extreme situations? Mothers lifting cars off their children, a Readers Digest sort of thing? The Guinness Book of World Records reported that Mrs. Maxwell Rogers lifted the end of a 3,600 pound truck off her son after a traffic accident. Compare that to the all time high world deadlift record of 925 pounds set by a 308 pound man!

Scientists speculate that in a life threatening situation your GTR could stop functioning. That gives you superhuman strength because your muscles don't shut down no matter how hard they pull. The fact that even in such circumstances people don't necessarily get injured says a lot about the true limitations of a human body.

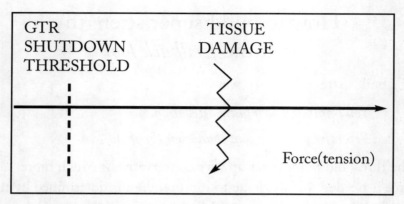

Repeatedly activating the GTR in training desensitizes it and raises your shutdown threshold. Your strength goes up—not to the degree of lifting cars, but enough to notice. And that is with a zero increase in muscle mass!

Plyometric stretching also disinhibits the GTR. It jerks on the tendons and if the jerk is quick, the GTR does not have the time to respond. Eventually it figures out, "Hey, I've been under such high tension and lived to tell about. Next time I will not bother to shut down the muscle, even if the force is applied slowly enough for me to respond."

Increase your strength by up to 20% with *Fascial Stretching* and *Digital Fascial Planing*

Another curious GTR disinhibiting technique is *fascial stretching*. Developed by East Coast bodybuilding consultant John Parrillo, it requires stretching a maximally pumped muscle past the point of pain and holding it for 10 seconds.

Fascia is that unappetizing fibrous sheath you trim off your steak before cooking it. Fascia surrounds and protects your muscles and other tissues. There are Golgi tendon organs in it, so it makes sense that stretching the fascia will desensitize them.

Pumping up the muscle beforehand serves to maximize the fascial stretch.

Parrillo claims strength increases of 20%. This seems a bit on the wild side, yet there is no doubt that the technique works. Isometrically stretching the pumped muscle should be even more effective than Parrillo's protocol.

John Parrillo also recommends *digital fascial planing*, stretching the fascia by having your training partner forcefully knead your pumped muscle with his or her second knuckle joints. The movement is linear, from the muscle's insertion towards its origin.

Three sets of twelve in the end of a weight training workout are recommended.

A potential benefit of both Parrillo's techniques is reduced risk of fascial hernias. Although fascia is stronger than structural steel at the molecular level, super tense muscle sometimes rips through it during extreme effort. I have a couple from holding on to heavy pulls like there was no tomorrow, odd looking bulges on my forearms where muscle had "spilled over."

It makes sense that stretched fascia—for the first time in this book I am talking about actual physical stretching—gives the muscles underneath more room to play. Still, most folks do not need to bother with fascial stretching. Fascial hernias are almost exclusively the domain of competitive powerlifters and arm wrestlers. Extreme tension of maximal lifts may pop the fascia, especially if the lifter ignores high rep muscle pumping that does stretch the fascia to a degree.

★

"My knees look like they lost a knife fight with a midget."

—E.J. Holub, former Kansas City Chiefs linebacker, on his 12 knee surgeries

★

The benefits, pitfalls, and limitations of full-range weight training. Flexibility vs. stability

Fitness glossies preach "full range" weight training as religiously as they preach the virtues of stretching. But is it necessary?

For the purpose of building extreme range strength, it is necessary, provided that:

> *the ligaments and tendons are not stretched*
>
> *you do not try to make your joints do the things our species was never designed to accomplish.*

We abuse our back, knees, and shoulders the most frequently. You may have seen, for instance, bodybuilders rounding their backs doing stiff legged dead lifts, trying to "get more stretch, man."

Or take the leg press (please!). People lower the weight till their knees touch their chests. Such range is impossible to achieve by movement in the hip joint alone, the spine has to flex, or round. The butt comes off the pad and the hundreds of pounds—even wimps usually can handle a couple times their body weight on the hip sled—are not distributed evenly over the surface of the back any more. The force is pointedly applied to one or two vertebrae and you had better be saving for a back surgery.

Knees also get screwed up a lot, especially the ligaments.

Ligaments hold your joints together. They do not stretch well, except in children. Stretch a ligament by only six percent and it will tear. Even if you manage to stretch it without tearing, do not consider yourself lucky. A stretched ligament means a loose, unstable, vulnerable joint, and a candidate for osteoarthritis.

It's time football coaches figured this one out. Did your coach

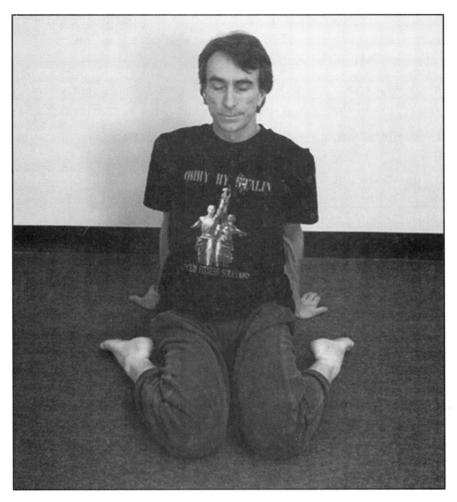

Stay away from this kind of stretch.

have you get down on your knees, sit back on your feet, and then have another player lean on your chest and push it as low as possible? Part of the game, right?

Well, your coach was a doorknob. This stretch made your knees weaker—and that is in a sport where knees are already at risk.

Ironically, according to Soviet research, stretching the ligaments is unnecessary even for the performance of most advanced gymnastic or martial arts skills. Even a suspended Chinese split can be achieved just by resetting the nervous regulation of muscular length and tension.

Your muscles have plenty of length to allow you to do splits, you just have to learn how to relax them.

While the splits, even a suspended wishbone, can be achieved with reeducating the nervous system, some Yoga asanas, the cow head pose and the frog pose, to name a couple, can only be performed by stretching the ligaments. Stay the hell away from them!

How can you tell if you are stretching a ligament?

If you feel discomfort or pain in the joint, then you are probably stretching the ligaments.

Women who are pregnant or had a child within a few months should be especially careful. Delivery of a child requires extraordinary flexibility and the woman's body releases the hormone *relaxin* to loosen the ligaments. Relaxin is not selective, ALL the ligaments are affected. They will not tear easily, but will stretch beyond the norm leading to joint instability.

Shoulders are another problem area. When you watch serious lifters and lightweights alike do dumbbell flies, dips, and the pec deck, it looks like they will not quit until their elbows touch behind the back. If these guys are wearing tank tops—and usually they are—you can see stretch marks on their shoulders. And those are the least of the problems of such training. Rotator cuff tears and ligament damage is worse.

Don't overstretch your shoulders. Do you really need more flexibility there? You do if you play baseball, but then you at least get paid for injuring yourself.

If you stop over stretching, can you keep doing the same lifting exercise for your pecs and shoulders?

Well, it depends on the individual. Some exercises are incompatible with certain physiques. For example, if I do parallel bar dips, my shoulders will be killing me for a week because I have a so-called separated A/C joint.

Dips, presses behind the neck, upright rows and flies are among such exercises. If an exercise aggravates your shoulders even with a light weight and a partial movement, don't count on being able to "work through" it. See a specialist and find a substitute.

If your shoulder problem comes from over stretched ligaments, you have to tighten the tissues around your shoulder, rather than stretch them.

Some of my victims started lifting with their shoulders in a very poor shape from old injuries. A light bench press would aggravate them, not to mention dips. But then, most of the time they could do a partial bench or an Olympic press in the rack with a respectable weight without as much as a twinge.

Yes, you lose some flexibility, but you gain stability. In Russia many people who would have gone under the knife in the States, are fixed up with limited range lifts. Something to think about.

Don't worry that you will not be able to develop "full muscle" with partials.

Although changing the exercise range or angle may alter the recruitment pattern, it is not going to develop some areas of the muscle more or less than others, thanks to *noncontiguous innervation.*

Each motor nerve controls its own group of muscle fibers called a *motor unit.* The constituent fibers are evenly spread out throughout the muscle, rather than being concentrated in its "peak," or "sweep," or any other part. So even if you manage to recruit a different motor unit, its fibers will still be all over the muscle.

Conclusion: it is impossible to change the shape of a muscle. A muscle is like a balloon—it will look different if you blow it up, but the inherent shape is still there. So do partials, and don't sweat it.

That does not mean though, that you cannot change the shape of a body part. You can—by focusing on different muscle groups and individual muscles within a muscle group. For example, emphasizing the short head of the biceps makes it "peaked" and overdeveloping the long head gives the biceps a more "stretched" look. But I'll save the details for another book.

How to develop functional strength using the Russian principle of *accentuation*

Full range strength training is the ticket for damage control, but not the best way to train for functional, usable strength.

Russian athletes follow the principle of *accentuation*. It means developing strength mostly in the range where high force output is required in one's sport. For example, a high jumper would emphasize partial, rather than full, squats because only the top few inches of the lockout are relevant to his sport.

★

"If they did [call me a sissy because I studied ballet], I'd stomp 'em and do a pirouette on their heads."

—Ken Avery, Cincinnati Bengals linebacker

★

Here is a quiz for you. Compare two athletes. One is a power-lifter who can full squat 500 pounds. He never did quarter squats and managed 600 when he tried it. This is a typical carryover, considering the obvious leverage advantage in the partial movement.

Another athlete, a high jumper, does quarter squats with 850 for reps, yet can full squat only 400. Who is stronger?

The typical response is "you are only as strong as your weak link." The weak link, or the "sticking point." in the squat is usually near the bottom or slightly above. Therefore, the conventional thinking goes, the jumper is weaker.

In an official powerlifting squat—yes. The rules say that your thighs must break the parallel. In a partial squat the jumper is 250 pounds stronger than the powerlifter. But it's a meaningless comparison. The high jumper does not compete in powerlifting and the powerlifter does not jump. For the high jump the sticking point on the bottom is irrelevant because the sport does not require you to squat so deep.

You can't compare apples and oranges.

Ironically, one of the strongest people I have stretched, an NFL player with an 800 full squat, was very weak in the extreme range of his hamstrings. Some of the ten-year-old ballerinas I have worked with pushed much harder in that range! Yet it did not stop the man from succeeding in his cutthroat sport. Specificity, again.

The weak link always progresses the slowest.

You will make much faster progress in the range of motion where you are at your strongest. An athlete with a 500 pound full squat and a 600 partial can build up to a parallel 600 and a partial 700 as a side effect in a couple of years, or work up to 800-1,000 pounds in the lockout in a fraction of the time.

Specificity is the key. It applies to every sport. If you are a football lineman and have to take off from a full squat, you've got to do full squats in training. A halfback, on the other hand, does not have to crouch and should focus on the partial squat.

A logical question is: wouldn't these partial lifts limit your flexibility? Yes, they would if you don't do some type of extreme range strength training, weights or isometrics. According to Dr. James Garrick, NFL medical advisor, this is what happened to football players when they started weight training in the sixties. Many got injured.

You know what happened next. Some Einstein came up with the idea that passively stretching the muscles before and after lifting would alleviate the problem. Ironically, about the same time the NFL switched to full range weight training. Injuries were reduced and it was incorrectly attributed to passive stretching.

No amount of passive stretching will compensate for resetting the stretch reflex at a shorter muscle length.

The nervous system adapts in response to strong stimuli. Compared to lifting weights, relaxed stretching is not intense enough to make an impact on it.

For instance, leg curls shorten the muscle because they overload the hamstrings in the contracted position. Toe touches and other relaxed stretches will NOT counteract this effect.

Instead you need to do another hamstring exercise that overloads the muscle in a stretched position—a stiff legged deadlift, for instance. It is important to do the exercises in that order. Of two stimuli of similar intensity, the last one is remembered better.

The moral of the story is not to kiss the partials goodbye, but rather to supplement them with extreme range strength training.

Your best bet is to emphasize partial lifts in your sport's functional range and throw in some longer-range exercises. For example, do quarter squats for 75% of your training plus full squats or lunges. Or complement the partials with isometric stretching.

How *Mobility Training* can save your joints and prevent or reduce arthritis

Osteoarthritis, a degenerative disease of joint cartilage, nails over 80% of people over sixty. You could be the next winner.

What does that have to do with stretching?

flexibility training improves your odds against arthritis.

If you already have arthritis, flexibility training will slow down the degenerative process and reduce the pain.

The type of flexibility training I am referring to is *mobility training*. This term was coined by Soviet scientist Nikolay Amosov, a public figure with the same stature in Russia as Arnold Schwarzenegger in this country.

You may be surprised to find out that the #1 Russian exercise icon is not a three hundred pound weightlifter, but an eighty-four year old surgeon with the wiry physique of a Bruce Lee and the ascetic fat free face of a Jacques Ives Cousteau.

Academician Nikolay Amosov runs a schedule that would a kill a twenty five year old yuppie, not to mention a horse. He performs two open heart surgeries a day, an average of eleven hours, wearing out a couple of crews of twenty year old nurses along the way. In his spare (?) time Amosov runs the Kiev Cardiovascular Surgery Institute of the Ukrainian Academy of Sciences, manages the famous Biocybernetics Department of the Ukrainian Academy of Sciences Cybernetics Institute and religiously follows his exercise regimen.

Nikolay Amosov has the biological age of forty. He looks it, he feels it, and a number of esoteric tests the Soviets are famous for have confirmed it.

Academician Amosov had not always been a human dynamo. The fitness superstar started out as a retired army lieutenant colonel in his late fifties with the World War Two behind him, a spare tire in the front, and an assortment of diseases. The turning point was the day when Amosov formulated and put into practice his now famous *theory of limit loads*.

One of the corner stones of the theory is the belief that a human organism has a great ability to regenerate itself. Use—intense use—is the key.

Orthopedics teaches that complete mobility of a joint is essential for its health.

Rotating a joint through its anatomically full range of motion— or trying to approach that range of motion if the joint is damaged—smoothes out the joint surfaces and improves the circulation. This contributes greatly to the joint's health.

Joint mobility is not the same as muscle flexibility. When doing mobility drills you usually do not feel much of a stretch, which is fine. A muscle does not always have to be stretched to put a joint through its full range of motion.

For example, in belly dancing the hip joints achieve almost the same range of motion as accomplished in a side split. Obviously, the "Elvis" is more practical than the "wishbone."

How much flexibility do you really need?

Is flexibility always good? Can you be too flexible?

Americans don't think so. They stretch just for the sake of stretching. They just can't get enough.

Sorry to burst your bubble. Soviet research demonstrated that you need only a small flexibility-reserve above the demands of your sport or activity. Excessive flexibility can actually be detrimental to athletic performance.

Old school strong men instinctively avoided stretching. They felt they could lift more weight by staying "tight." They were right. The stretch reflex fired sooner, making them more prone to an injury, but helping them to move more iron.

Russian Olympic weightlifters avoid full range movements of the muscles surrounding the hip and knee joints. Too much flexibility in those areas makes the lifter sink too deep when he is getting under the barbell.

The same is true in powerlifting. Fortunately, powerlifters, as a group, are the least influenced by our pop fitness culture's deification of relaxed stretching, high-carb/low fat/low protein diet, and other stupid ideas. Dr. Judd says that "it would probably be easier to find a legitimate television evangelist than a power-lifter who can touch his toes without bending his knees." Big fat hairy deal.

That is not to say that powerlifters do not need flexibility. They do—but no more than necessary to lift with good form. For example, tight hamstrings "tuck your butt in." As a result, back strength is wasted on fighting against your own hams, rather than the weight in the squat and deadlift.

★

"We did it for Britain and for the hell of it."

—Richard Noble, on breaking the world automobile speed record

★

Soviet researcher and weightlifting coach R. A. Roman determined that an athlete loses fifteen percent of his deadlifting strength when he pulls with a rounded, rather than a flat back. That could mean the difference between the first and last place!

Also, your hamstrings or back are likely to get injured. Hamstrings take forever to heal, but it is not the end of the world. The back is a more serious matter. A properly arched spine can support 10 times more weight than a straight one. Rounding your back makes it even more vulnerable. Ever heard a disk blow out? Sounds like a high tension cable going boink!

The lesson is not to stretch your hams until you can tie your shoes with your teeth, but just enough to maintain a tight arch in the "hole"—the bottom of the squat.

Never compensate for poor technique with flexibility.

Bodybuilders often complain how limited ankle flexibility affects their squat. Sorry, boys, when you squat properly, the movement in the ankle is minimal and you should be able to squat wearing ski boots. Learn to squat from a powerlifter and do not waste your time in a ballet class.

It applies to every sport. Be just a touch more flexible than you have to be. You must be sick of powerlifting examples by now, so I'll switch the tune.

In sprinting an excessively loose trunk prevents one from maximally exploiting the pumping action of the arms. In shot put or boxing a super flexible waist will absorb the drive from the legs instead of transferring it to the shoulder. Etcetera, etcetera.

Generally, you need only a small reserve of flexibility beyond the requirements of your sport—or your lifestyle.

In my seminars I often hear people say, "I want to be able to touch my toes."

"Why?" I ask. "Does the inability to do it prevent you from doing anything?"

"No," they reply, "I just know I am supposed to be able to do it."

Don't let the media tell you what you are supposed and not supposed to do. Unless your tight hamstrings affect your spinal alignment, your sport requires you to bend over and touch your toes, don't sweat it.

The fact that the sit-and-reach is a part of the standard flexibility test is meaningless. Flexibility is highly specific—in speed, the joints tested, and even the body position.

That is why standard flexibility tests, like the NFL's sit-and-reach test, are worthless. I once showed a Tampa Bay Buccaneer how to cheat on it because it is as relevant to his ability on the football field as a chess gambit.

My sit-and-reach is below average—I can barely touch my toes. Yet I do splits with ease. It makes sense. I train the splits and do not bother with the sit-and-reach.

It's about credibility. Thanks to Jean Claude Van Damme, everybody thinks it is cool when you hang suspended between chairs. When I tore a knee ligament and could not do my demonstrations for a couple of months, people who attended my seminars weren't nearly as pumped as they used to be. It's an MTV thing. Americans are more impressed with what they see, than what they hear.

The "show me!" attitude is not limited to Missouri. And often it's easier to show than to explain that a nice smile does not make a person an expert in dental care. So as much as I hate splits, and as little as I need them, I keep splitting. The things we do for money!

Although I have less than average genetic potential to do the sit-and-reach, my flexibility will be off the charts in a couple of months if I apply the shutdown threshold isometrics to this exercise. But the fact that the splits did not affect the sit-and-reach, teaches one important lesson: flexibility is position specific.

Flexibility developed with one exercise does not always improve the range of motion of the same joint when tested in other exercises.

In one study a group of subjects trained the toe-reach standing, and the other trained while seated. Those who stretched in the seated position did not do well when they were tested standing. The other group did well on both tests. Go figure.

Conclusion: the transfer of training effect is inconsistent. Sometimes you have it, sometimes you don't. If a stretching exercise does not improve your sport's functional flexibility—ditch it.

It goes without saying that improving flexibility in one joint does not make you more flexible in others. The sit-and-reach will do diddly for your shoulder flexibility.

To sum up: stretch barely beyond the requirements of your sport or lifestyle. Very few athletes need to be hyperflexible. So I'll either teach you how to do splits, or will talk you out of it.

Part Two: Do It My Way

Effective mobility training for your joints

Mobility training involves making slow circles with your joints, starting with small amplitude and working up to the joint's maximum range.

Mobility drills are ideally performed every morning. You will not only do your joints a favor, but will get rid of stiffness as well.

You get "rusty" whenever your *proprioceptors*—the sensors that give your body information about its position in space, its speed of movement etc.—do not get any new input for awhile.

When nothing happens, your nervous system is not sure what to expect from the environment and tightens your muscles—just in case. That's why you feel like the Tin Man in the morning or after any long period of inactivity.

Movement wakes up your proprioceptors, the nervous system chills out and you limber up. More important, mobility training increases the blood flow to the joints, lubricates them, and keeps their surfaces smooth and healthy. A full range of motion is gained and maintained.

Do your mobility drills until your joints are rolling smoothly and additional exercise does not make any difference. Or do as many repetitions as your age.

Older joints need more movement. For damaged joints work up to 300 rotations. You can do them in one or more sets depending on your preference and endurance.

Attention, wimps who insist on warming up before every exercise bout! Mobility training happens to warm you up, so why don't you do it instead of riding your stationary bike? At least you will not be wasting time. It is not much different from what Russian ballet dancers do.

You tough cookies who had the will power to quit warmups, should do the joint exercises only in the morning.

It is most convenient to do your mobility drills and dynamic stretches together, in that order. The distinction is not always clear. While some exercises are pure joint mobility drills or muscle stretches, others, like the side to side neck tilts, are combinations. Because these two types of exercises are not done the same way, differentiate whenever possible.

Mobility drills are always done slowly, with complete control. Dynamic stretches will eventually become very fast.

The optimal sequence for both types of exercises is from the extremities towards the center. They are listed in that order.

Effective dynamic flexibility training for the muscles

When you are done with joint rotations, move on to dynamic flexibility exercises for the muscles associated with that joint.

Start with complete control, no bounce and a limited range of motion. Gradually increase the range and speed, both in the context of one workout and the entire training cycle.

You will make most of your progress in two to three months. At the end of this period you should have enough flexibility for most sports and be able to display it at your sport's velocity. If your joints are the limiting factor, it may take longer. Emphasize mobility training to reshape their surfaces.

IMPORTANT: the idea of dynamic flexibility training is NOT to force a muscle into a new range by building up momentum.

Performed as described it WILL set off the stretch reflex and the slip on ice scenario will follow.

When my dad took up winter swimming, a popular Russian sport, he did not jump into the ice hole the first time round. That would have guaranteed pneumonia.

No, Vladimir Tsatsouline started swimming in July and practiced daily. Water temperature was dropping by a fraction of a point each day, giving the body a chance to adapt. By the time December rolled around, my dad got desensitized to cold water. Thanks to this gradual approach, this year the old man won the White Russian Nationals!

So, a properly performed dynamic stretch is terminated RIGHT BEFORE the stretch reflex fires. As a result, the reflex threshold will move up and next time you will be able to move a little further and faster.

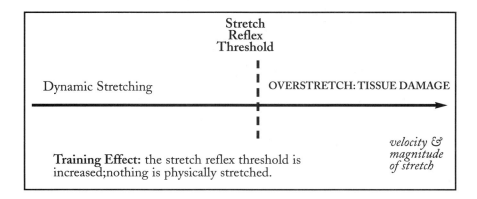

Dynamic/plyometric stretches should be done two to seven days a week for as many sets as it takes to achieve your maximal amplitude for the day—*but no more*.

Too many repetitions in the same range will solidify the memory of how far your muscle can be stretched. It will be hard to break it and establish new levels of flexibility in later workouts. Advanced athletes will only need one set.

Stretch in sets of five to fifteen repetitions. Avoid getting tired. Fatigued muscles are less elastic and you will defeat the purpose of your training.

One exception is the development of dynamic flexibility endurance. Kickboxers, for instance, need to keep up their kicks for up to twelve rounds.

But even if it applies to you, don't do flexibility endurance drills until you have developed your flexibility to the top level required in your sport.

Effective plyometric flexibility training

The same applies to plyometric flexibility drills. Work on the height and speed of your kicks bounce free. Only when they are satisfactory, go ballistic.

"Ballistic" does NOT mean letting the momentum tear your muscles.

Correct plyometric flexibility training entails:

moving at the maximum velocity you can still control

and quickly reversing the stretch precisely at the point where your stretch reflex fires—not sooner (standard dynamic stretching), or later (injury).

Dynamic Stretching	vs.	**Plyometric Stretching**
Complete control, no momentum		Ballistic
Movement smoothly reversed right before the stretch reflex fires		Movement sharply reversed when the stretch reflex fires
		Emphasis on touch and go. NOTA BENE!: no further stretch after the reflex is set off!

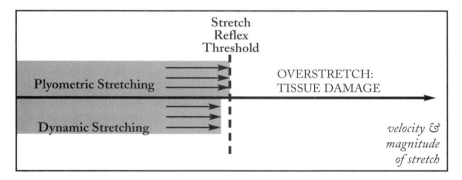

Plyometric exercises performed to improve immediate athletic performance should be similar in form and range to the event. For instance, martial artists should do plyometric kicks, jump squats are the thing for Alpine skiers, and the best bet for runners is the Russian lunge, a bouncy lunge with a quick switch of legs.

Complex training and powerlifting applications

The plyometric/weight lifting sequence is called *complex training*. Its effect goes beyond immediate performance. Because you end up lifting more weight, you will become stronger. It applies not only to competitive powerlifters, but to anybody training with weights.

Specific guidelines for powerlifting applications were developed by Dr. Fred "Squat" Hatfield, one of the most competent sports scientists on this side of what used to be the Iron Curtain and the first man to officially squat 1,000 pounds.

For the dead lift Dr. "Squat" recommends doing one or two explosive vertical jumps right before the attempt. He warns that the effect is lost if the lifter spends too much time adjusting his grip.

Since the hips and back, rather than the thighs, do most work in the dead lift, I believe that the jump is not the best exercise for increasing your immediate dead lift performance.

I propose the one arm snatch.

This exercise is a part of the kettlebell lifting competition, a popular ethnic Russian strength sport. Since you cannot buy a "kettlebell," a big metal ball with a handle, in the US, a dumbbell will do.

Use a light dumbbell. It will not feel light because of the momentum it is going to build up.

Press the dumbbell over your head and spread your feet slightly wider than your shoulders.

Inhale, arch your back, and let the dumbbell free fall between your legs, at the same time pushing your hips back. Make sure the weight falls as close to your body as possible. Stay on your heels.

Once the dumbbell reaches the bottom position, without hesitation explosively lift it overhead. Don't try to lift it with your arm and shoulder—rather drive your hips through. You might get airborne. It is OK.

Repeat three times with each arm.

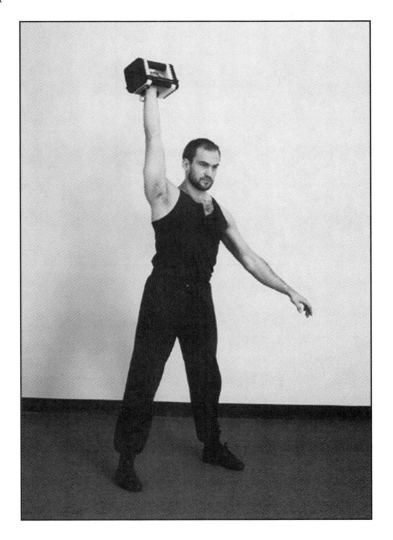

One-arm snatch

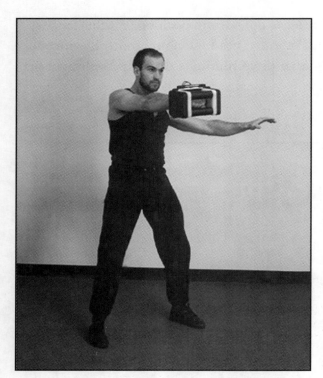

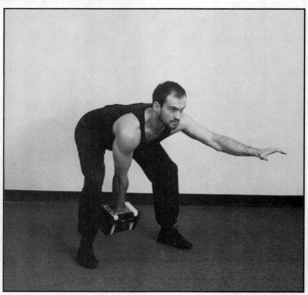

For the bench press the obvious solution of lowering the bar very fast is not a good one. You might get red lights from the judges for bouncing the bar or beating the clap, and could crush your rib cage. Instead, Dr. Hatfield recommends violently throwing your elbows back a few times right before the hand off. Once again, don't screw around with the hand off and descent, or the effect will be lost.

For the squat Dr. Hatfield suggests a modified "dive-bomb squat." The conventional dive-bomb squat involves a free fall into the "hole" and is popular among superheavyweights. Unless you have calves the size of an average waist and a huge gut to rebound from, your knees are in trouble.

Dr. Hatfield modified the dive-bomb squat by lowering the weight under control, then free falling only the last one or two inches. It is safer and it works.

Another trick Hatfield used with the squat was preceding the attempt with either vertical jumps, like for the deadlift, or depth jumps.

Depth jumps are a form of plyometrics. Step off a 30-40" bench and drop straight down. The moment you hit the ground, forcefully rebound straight up, spending as little time as possible in transition. A useful image is jumping on a hot stove.

Land on the balls of your feet, followed by the whole feet. Don't bend your legs more than necessary. Use a resilient surface, such as a gymnastic mat, or grass.

Martial arts applications

In addition to dynamic/plyometric and isometric stretching, martial artists need a couple of specialized conditioning techniques. I'll call them "hand kicking" and "shaking out" for the lack of nerdier terms.

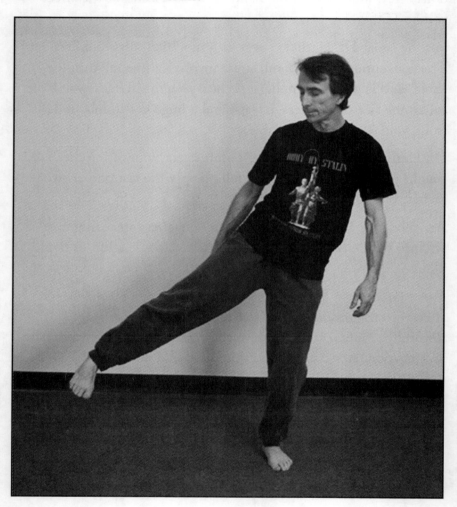

"Shakeouts."

"Shaking out" is not a form of stretching, but a tendon and ligament strengthening method. It prepares you for the time when the target isn't there.

Have you ever walked down dark stairs with one step too many?

I bet your knee did not appreciate you stepping into space expecting to meet the solid ground. The same thing happens when an over committed thrust kick misses its target—your knee's connective tissues absorb the impact.

It is logical to strengthen them.

Weight training could do that, but most leg exercises—the squat, for instance—condition you against compression, rather than extension. The only exercise I can think of that does the job is the reverse squat in gravity boots. The problem with it is almost unavoidable lower back damage—ask your chiropractor for details.

A "shakeout" is a snap kick of any variety—front, side, hook, or roundhouse—in the air, without pullout.

Keep your muscles maximally relaxed to let the knee hyperextend and absorb the shock. It should feel like you are trying to "throw away" the part of your leg from the knee down, or kick a shoe off your foot.

Get into this form of conditioning very gradually, with very light snaps, as there is considerable risk of an injury. Still, it is worth it. Your odds against causing more serious damage when a committed kick fails to connect with your opponent will improve. Over a period of time controlled jerks on the tendons and ligaments will make them thicker and stronger.

Do not abuse this method. Connective tissues adapt to stress slowly. Limit your "shakeout" workouts to a few times a month, always place them last in a practice, after sparring and conditioning.

Shakeouts can develop bad kicking habits. To avoid negative transfer follow them up with a couple of perfect kicks on a heavy bag—with proper tightening on the impact and well timed pullout.

"Hand kicking" is a form of dynamic stretching for the legs that requires your hand to stop a fast moving leg. It conditions you to have the maximal speed in your kicks even near the limits of your flexibility.

It is hard to develop because your nervous body does not feel safe when a leg is moving away at a high speed. It builds up a lot of momentum and the nervous system realizes that something might get hurt unless it puts a stop to it.

The stretch reflex clicks in. The hamstrings and groin muscles of both legs start contracting long before you are at full extension to have a chance at stopping the runaway leg. If it happens suddenly, you will pull a muscle. If gradually—the kick will "brake" before the impact. Both scenarios are unacceptable.

Hand kicks will train your stretch reflex not to fire even at maximal speed and near the limit of your flexibility. It works for the same reason you can touch your nose in the dark. Your nervous system knows that your hand is there to stop the fast moving leg and will not activate the stretch reflex.

Pneumomuscular flexibility training

Warning!

Many American physicians believe that holding your breath during exercise could be hazardous to your health. If you have a heart problem, high blood pressure, or other health concerns, consult your physician before attempting the breathing patterns described in this book.

Get in the position of a comfortable stretch, placing most of your weight on the muscles you are stretching.

Inhale maximally and tighten up your entire body, especially the target muscles.

Deepest relaxation can be only achieved with a contrast with greatest tension—the ying and yang of stretching, so to say. Think of your body as a fist. Making fists helps. Pay attention not to decrease the amount of stretch when you are tightening up!

Hold your breath—and tension—for a couple of seconds, the suddenly let all the tension out with a sigh of relief. Let your jaw and shoulders go limp with the rest of your body.

Visualize transforming from a tight spring into a limp noodle in a blink of an eye. A burst balloon is another useful analogy. Or try this vivid description of the tension/release sequence by Dr. Judd Biasiotto: "You must relax instantly. To better illustrate what it would feel like to "turn off" as you have been instructed, picture yourself exerting all your strength in an effort to push a large boulder off a sheer cliff. When suddenly the boulder goes over the edge, there is no active resistance to your pushing and all you straining instantly ceases. It is that feeling, that nothingness after the boulder drops, that you are striving to obtain when you "turn off your source of power."

At this point the stretch will increase as the involved body parts will drop down when the tension is released. Don't let them drop more than an inch or so at a time to make your stretches safer.

Keep repeating the drill until you can no longer increase your range of motion. Do as many sets as it takes to reach your maximal flexibility for the day—but no more! Stretch one to two times a week, never before activities requiring much exertion or coordination.

★

"Have the strength to force the moment to its crisis."

—Thomas Stearns Eliot

★

Shutdown threshold isometric flexibility training

First, write a will.

Then stretch as far as you comfortably can.

Next, contract the target muscles, as if trying to reverse the stretch.

Start pushing gently and build up the tension to the max over a few seconds. Remember, it is the sudden combination of stretch and contraction that causes most injuries!

If you are lucky, your super tense muscles will collapse, like your biceps going jello when you get beat in arm wrestling. If it does not happen, and it might take you awhile to get the hang of it, you have two options:

> 1. Keep pushing. Eventually, in a couple of painful minutes at the most, the exhausted muscles will collapse. The harder and steadier you push, the sooner they will go, and you want that because isometric stretching isn't fun.

Do NOT lighten up the pressure when it becomes unbearable! Not even for a second! If you do, you are only going to get exhausted, not flexible. Tough it out. I never promised it would be easy.

If you have a hard time understanding what you are supposed to feel, lower yourself in a pushup position—on your knees if standard pushups are too difficult—and stop with your chest half an inch above the ground.

Hold that position for as long as you can, until you literally collapse on the floor.

> 2. If you faithfully followed the instructions and the muscle still hasn't buckled in in a couple of painful minutes, fake it by relaxing it exactly as you have done when you practiced pneumomuscular stretching.

Sigh with relief, and eke out a little more stretch. Don't force it, especially those of you who are "almost there" in the splits.

You can increase the range of motion with the help of gravity, or by contracting the muscles that oppose the ones you are stretching. For example, you can recruit the quads against the hamstrings. We call these opposing muscle groups antagonists.

Antagonistic contraction will not only move your limbs further, but will relax the target muscles even more, thanks to reciprocal inhibition.

It is all about efficiency. When one muscle is working, its antagonist on the other side of the joint relaxes so it does not act as a brake.

Never do STI stretches with a partner! The pressure must be released the moment your GTR fires, and sooner or later a knockout blonde will walk by and your buddy will miss the moment. You are the only person who can get the timing right.

How can you push against yourself? With the help of gravity.

You just have to be careful about how much weight you put on the target muscle.

Here is a horror scenario:

Imagine doing a suspended isometric side split with your hands in the air—and an extra weight that triggers a reflexive contraction of your groin muscles, without any effort on your part.

The GTR fires and you drop deeper. The stretch reflex will try to fire to stop you but will be overridden by the GTR that has seniority in the reflex hierarchy. You will be falling deeper and deeper, building up momentum along the way and ripping yourself in half.

Are you scared? Good. Now here is what you should do:

Pick stretches where it takes the COMBINED EFFORTS OF GRAVITY AND YOURS to generate enough tension for a shutdown.

You can either vary the body position, or even shift some of your weight on your arms if you do a split, for instance.

~~GRAVITY = SHUTDOWN LEVEL TENSION~~
GRAVITY + WILLFUL CONTRACTION =
SHUTDOWN LEVEL TENSION

Contract the target muscles maximally and the GTR will fire. You will drop an inch or two, and the stretch reflex will take over. Your muscles will tense again and stop you before you have built up too much momentum. You can catch yourself with your arms too.

Now, YOU can decide when the GTR should fire again— whenever you contract your muscles at will.

Don't get defensive though. You have to apply enough force for the GTR to fire. Otherwise, the stretch will not work. You will get tired, that's all.

Because an STI contraction typically takes longer than a brief pneumomuscular one, you should not be holding your breath when you push. However, you want your muscles to be tense continuously, and it is impossible when you breathe normally. The compromise is to breathe very frequently, but shallow. Breathe as if you do not want anybody to hear that you are breathing. Keep your abs tight and don't hyperventilate. When you release the tension, breathe normally. It will help you relax.

Repeat the contract/relax sequence until your stretch stops increasing. Rest for a couple of minutes, shaking and loosening up the target muscles, and do another set.

For the easily stretched muscles in the upper body you are unlikely to ever need STI; one set of PFT is usually enough. Two to five sets of STI usually hit the spot for the back and legs. If your muscles are sore and/or you cannot achieve the same level of stretch as in the previous set, you have overdone it. Next workout subtract one set.

The following schedule works well for most people:

Do two sets progressively more intense sets of pneumomuscular stretching. When you cannot increase the stretch without a Golgi tendon shutdown, relax and stay in that position for a minute.

Start the third set with short (3-5 seconds), powerful contractions. Get to the level of stretch achieved in the last set without delay, and start STI. Now the duration of each contraction is as long as it takes for the Golgi tendon reflex to fire. At this point don't hold back. The harder you push, the sooner the muscle will shut down!

Once you have achieved your maximal flexibility for the day, contract the stretched muscles hard and hold the tension for up to 30 seconds. It is tougher than ten miles of detour! Don't forget to breathe.

If you hit a plateau, stop trying to increase the range for awhile. Instead, concentrate on building strength. Remember that your nervous system is more willing to let you have a range of motion that you can control. Push harder. Push longer.

Even if you are not at a standstill, near the end of the stretch— where the going gets tough—it is a good idea not to increase the range after every contraction. Try every second or third contraction.

Shutdown threshold isometrics mess with your proprioceptors and impair your coordination for the rest of the day. So don't do them before your sport practice. Do them last. The rule of thumb is: if you have to do an isometric stretch before you engage in your sport, you are not ready for the skill you are practicing. There are very few exceptions. For example, shoulder and wrist isometrics before squats for the lifters who cannot get under the bar otherwise.

Don't do isometrics too often. Treat them as strength exercises that they are. One or two sessions a week are optimal. Three times in two weeks, for example Monday, Friday, then Wednesday of the next week, also works well.

It gets better. The more advanced you are, the less of it you need. Once you have mastered the tension and length control it is hard to lose it. I maintain my flexibility with only two to three isometric stretching sessions a month, one set each. I can do splits and high kicks cold. You can too.

Mike Song, a rock climber who did a split a couple of weeks after he took my seminar, was too busy to train for a month afterwards. To his surprise he went all the way into a full split the first time he tried it after a layoff! In fact, occasional layoffs of a week or two will help you to improve due to the *reminiscence effect*.

In 1984 Jerry Moffat, the world's top dog rock climber, called it quits and rode into the sunset on his motorcycle. Nobody expected miracles from Jerry when he came back to the rock two years later. Yet two weeks after his comeback the man climbed the best performance of his career!

Motor learning people know that a skill tends to improve after a lay-off. It is called the reminiscence effect.

Multiple repetition of a movement, a rock climbing technique, or the squat, forms what Russians call the *dynamic stereotype,* or a "how to manual" of this movement in the athlete's brain. You learn to perform it exactly as practiced—the form, the force, the range of motion, etc.

Although forming a dynamic stereotype is necessary to master a sports skill, once it is formed, it is difficult to improve on. Once you have reached a plateau, continued practice only reinforces it.

If you lay off stretching, your brain gets a chance to forget your limit. This is the essence of the reminiscence effect. Once your old PR has been erased, you are ready to train for a new one!

Stretching when injured

Rehabilitation is not my area of expertise. Over the years I have learned to talk only about the things that I know something about, so I'll keep it brief. I will also limit my rehab advice to muscle tears—everything else is your doctor's problem.

In one sentence, RICE it, then stretch it. I will not babble about RICE because everybody else does. On to stretching.

Do it—ASAP, certainly within 24 hours. When a muscle tears, so do blood vessels. Internal bleeding causes the muscle to contract, a typical reaction to any foreign matter.

Whenever it hits the fan, muscles retreat into spasm—just in case. This creates a couple of problems:

First, healing takes forever. High muscle tension restricts circulation. This may be a useful feature immediately after the injury to keep the swelling down, but it becomes counterproductive after a day or two.

Second, as a result of limited blood supply and inactivity, the muscle atrophies.

And third, flexibility is lost. When a muscle spends a lot of time in a shortened position, the stretch reflex is down-regulated. A shorter muscle length and higher tension become the norm.

A weaker and tighter muscle will lead to more problems down the line. It is likely to get reinjured, and so are healthy muscles, as a result of imbalance or compensation.

So stretch the damn thing! Find whatever hurts the most and do it, stopping just short of PAIN, in caps. Rehab is a cliche business—no pain, no gain.

Pneumomuscular stretching is very effective in relieving tension, regardless of its source. A form of strength training, it also helps to prevent muscle atrophy. Do it many times throughout the day.

Keep in mind that stretching is not a panacea, especially for the back.

Those of you with bad backs—and if statistics don't lie, it's every other American—note on your forehead:

stretching will relieve the pain, but will not fix you up.

Spasms and pain are only symptoms. The real problem is usually weakness.

A weak back muscle has to contract hard just to keep you from walking on all fours—spinal erectors are "anti-gravity muscles." The contraction is difficult to maintain, so the muscle just locks. Movement and circulation become limited, so it gets even weaker—so it cramps even more to get even weaker to cramp even more… It's a vicious circle.

Conclusion: Trying to fix a bad back with stretching is about as useful as an oil change on the *Titanic.* You'd better get on a first name basis with deadlifts. Ab strength is also very important. Check out my new book *Beyond Crunches: Hard Science. Hard Abs.*

The New Flexibility Commandments

■ Only a small flexibility reserve is needed beyond the needs of one's sport or activity. Excessive flexibility can be detrimental to performance in many sports.

■ Extreme flexibility can be obtained at any age without changing the mechanical properties of your tissues. The key is resetting the nervous control of muscular length and tension.

■ Flexibility is speed specific, therefore dynamic flexibility training is a must. Dynamic stretching isn't 100% safe. Nothing is.

■ There isn't such a thing as "injury prevention"—only "damage control."

■ A muscle does not have to be maximally stretched to be torn. A combination of a sudden stretch and contraction does it.

■ In high force accidents flexibility becomes a liability, unless the individual is very strong in the extreme range of motion.

■ An optimal flexibility training regimen involves: mobility training to keep the joints from being the limiting factor; pneumomuscular stretching; isometric flexibility training to develop extreme range; and dynamic flexibility training which will allow you to have that range with speed. Relaxed stretching belongs on the junk pile of history next to communism.

Part Three: Mobility Drills and Dynamic Stretches

Make sure to carefully study the fine points of dynamic stretching in Part II before doing the following exercises!

Some exercises, for example shoulder rolls, are pure mobility drills. They are marked **[M]**. Others are pure stretches, marked **[F]**. The distinction is important because these exercises are done differently. Mobility drills are always done slowly, with complete control. Dynamic stretches will eventually become very fast. Sets and repetitions also vary, as you remember.

If a drill is a combination **[MF]**, perform it as a stretch, but make sure to do the first set slowly.

The neck and some back exercises were not designated **[MF]**, because performing them rapidly could injure the spine. The risk to benefit ratio is not good.

PHOTOS

Mobility Drills & Dynamic Stretches

1. Neck flexion/extension [M]
2. Neck lateral flexion [M]
3. Neck rotation [M]
4. Shoulder rolls [M]
5. Wrist circles [M]
6. Fist [MF]
7. Elbow circles [M]
8. Arm circles [MF]
9. Vertical arm swings *(shoulder girdle)* [F]
10. Horizontal arm swings *(shoulder girdle)* [F]
11. "Scarecrow" *(rotator cuffs)* [F]
12. Archer stretch *(lats and triceps)* [F]
13. Lateral spine flexion [MF]
14. Spine rotation [M]
15. Forward spine flexion [MF]
16. Spine extension [M]
17. Toe fist [MF]
18. Ankle rotation [M]
19. Knee circles [M]
20. Hoola hoop [M]
21. Belly dancing [M]
22. Squats [M]
23. Stair calf stretch [F]
24. Front hand kick *(hamstrings)* [F]
25. Side hand kick *(inner thighs: hip adductors)* [F]
26. Outside crescent hand kick *(inner thighs: internal hip rotators)* [F]
27. Inside crescent hand kick *(outer thighs: hip abductors, external hip rotators)*
28. Butt kicks *(quads)* [F]
29. Lunge *(hip flexors)* [F]

Isometric and Extreme Range Stretches

30. Neck forward flexion
31. Neck lateral flexion
32. Neck rotation
33. Wrist flexion
34. Wrist extension
35. Doorway stretch
36. Table top lat stretch
37. Archer stretch *(lats and triceps)*
38. Crossover stretch *(upper back, midback & back of the shoulders)*
39. Toe extension
40. Standing calf stretch *(gastrocnemius)*
41. Seated calf stretch *(soleus)*
42. "Pretzel" *(spine rotation & outer thighs: hip abductors)*
43. Hamstring towel stretch
44. Hamstring chair stretch
45. Toe touch *(hamstrings, glutes & lower back)*
46. Powerlifter's back and hamstring stretch
47. Spine decompression
48. Spine extension
49. Low back stress hip flexor stretch
50. Hip flexor & quad stretch
51. Front split
52. Hip flexor glute & outer thigh stretch
53. Internal hip rotator & hip flexor stretch
54. Groin stretch #1
55. Groin stretch #2
56. Wall split
57. (Suspended) side split

Stretches with weights

58. Stiff-legged deadlift *(right & wrong)*
59. Spider lift
60. Overhead squat

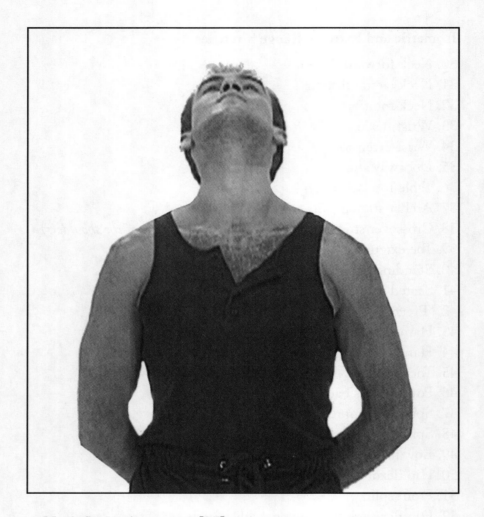

1. Neck flexion/extension [M]

Slowly tilt your head back as far as it comfortably goes, while trying to sort of "elongate" your neck, then tuck your chin in as much as possible.

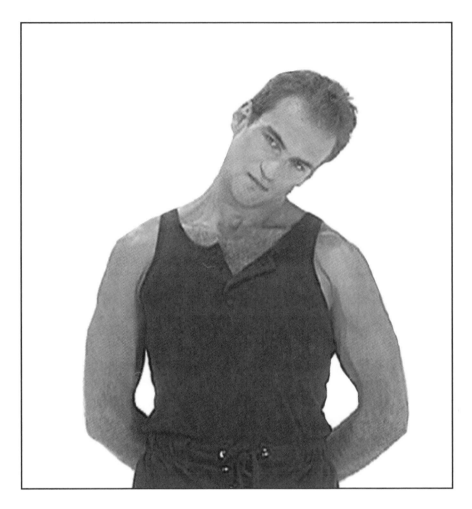

2. Neck lateral flexion [M]

Tilt your head to one side as far as possible,
then the other side. Move strictly, no twisting!

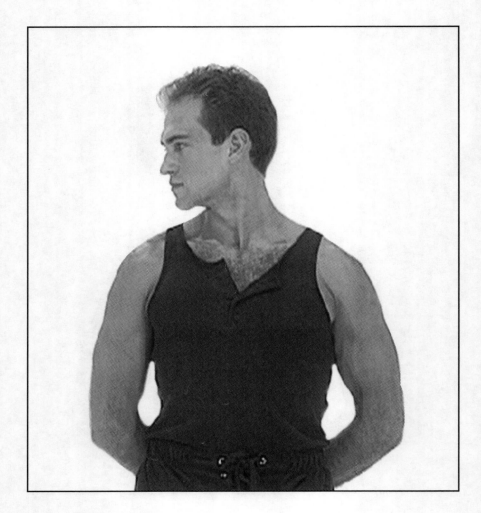

3. Neck rotation [M]

Slowly rotate your head left, then right.
Again, no twisting!

You might ask, why do three separate neck movements
if I can cover all the bases with a neck roll?

The answer is, it could damage your cervical spine.

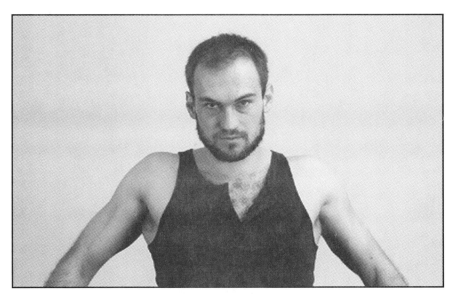

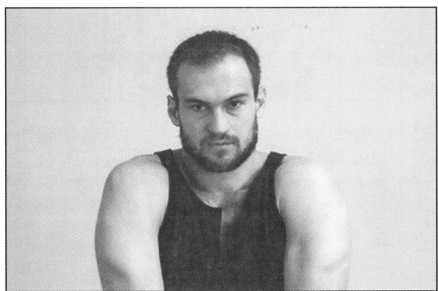

4. Shoulder rolls [M]

Roll your shoulders back and forth with maximal amplitude. Feel free to change the direction whenever you like.

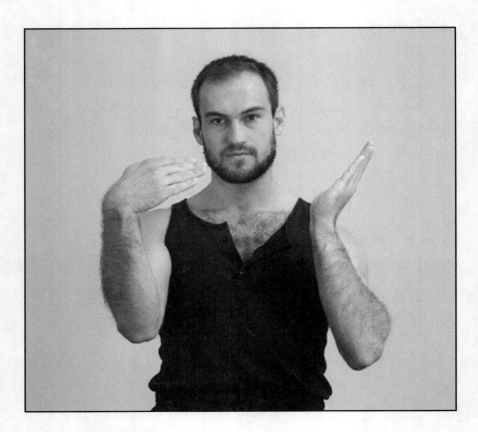

5. Wrist circles [M]

Make circles with your wrists while holding your
fingers straight and together—although not tight.

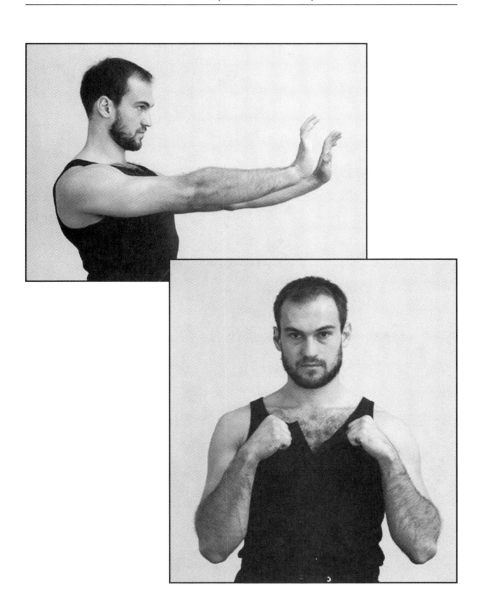

6. Fist [MF]

Make loose fists while keeping your elbows bent, then open them while straightening out your arms and pulling your fingers back as far as possible.

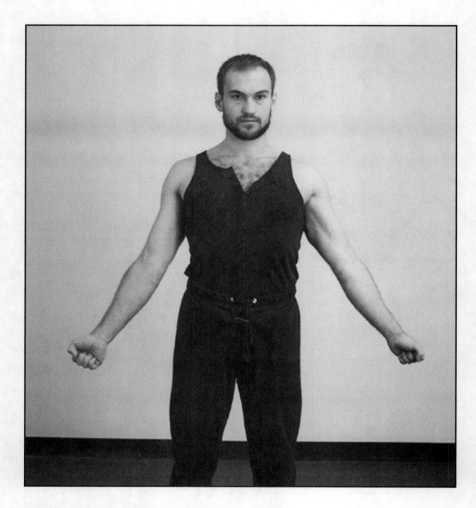

7. Elbow circles [M]

Tuck your elbows into your sides and make circles with
your forearms. The movement is like a dumbbell curl with
a circle.

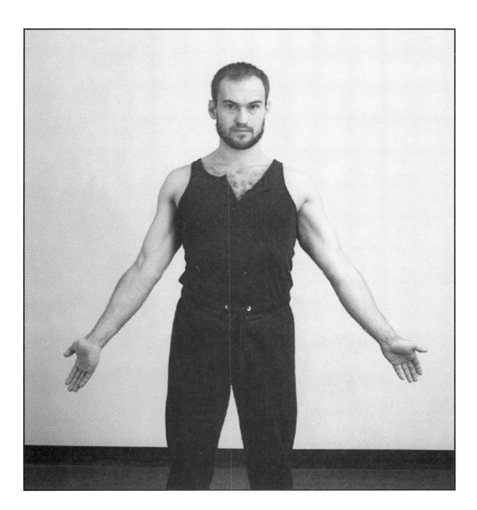

8. Arm circles [MF]

Make circles with your arms. Start small and gradually increase the amplitude. Feel free to change the direction any time.

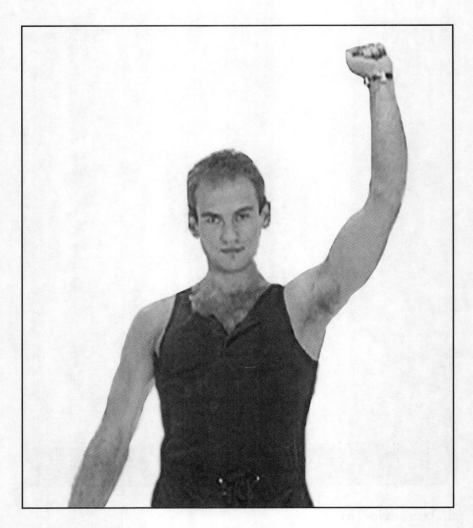

9. Vertical arm swings *(shoulder girdle)* **[F]**

Make loose fists. Raise one arm and bring both arms back twice, then switch.

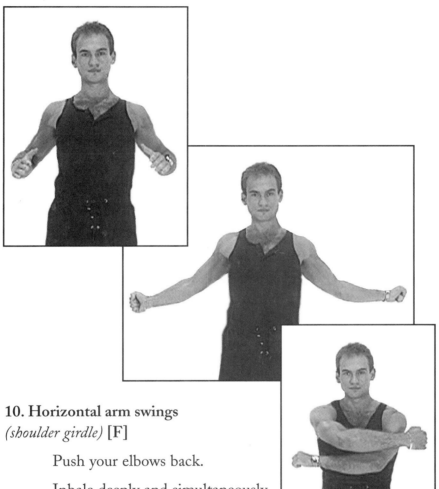

10. Horizontal arm swings
(shoulder girdle) **[F]**

Push your elbows back.

Inhale deeply and simultaneously stretch your arms back as if you are a bow. Imagine that I put my foot between your shoulder blades and pull on your arms. As in the previous drill, the "one-two" count works well

Exhale, letting your rib cage shrink and your back slump. At the same time sort of hug yourself. Shall we call this the "Saturday Night Live Stretch"?

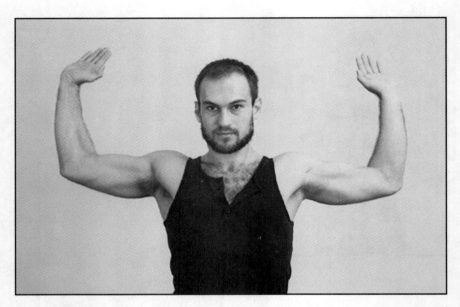

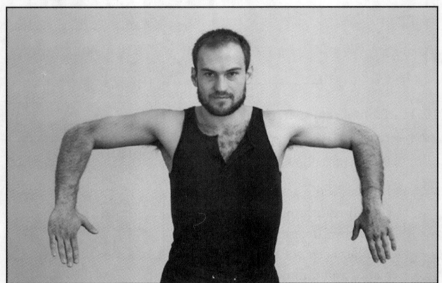

11. "Scarecrow" *(rotator cuffs)* [F]

It's Halloween and you are dressed up as a scarecrow! You have a broomstick for shoulders and you are trying to rotate your arms around it.

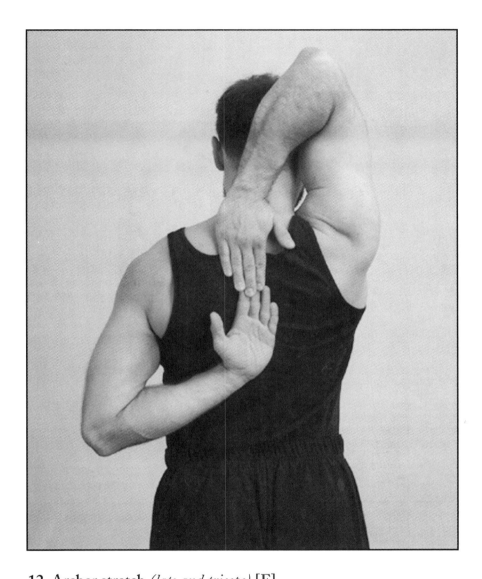

12. Archer stretch *(lats and triceps)* [F]

Try to meet your hands behind your back. Don't stop
or twist your torso.

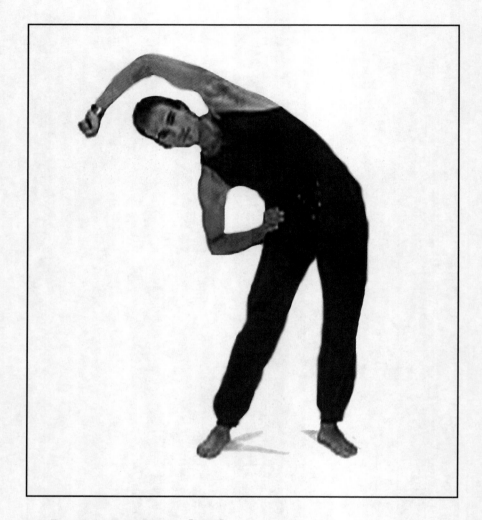

13. Lateral spine flexion [MF]

Bend sideways—strictly sideways.

No twisting!

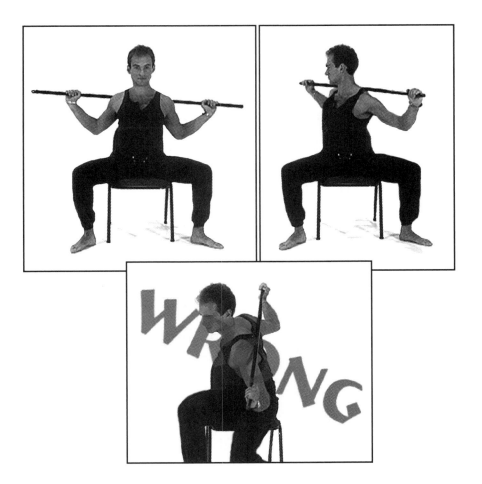

14. Spine rotation [M]

Sit in a chair with your feet planted wide and solid.
That is supposed to immobilize your hips.

Hold a broomstick on your shoulders and keep your back
upright and chest out. The broomstick helps to eliminate
the movement of the shoulders and concentrate on your
spine.

Look up and twist. Nothing is supposed to move from
the waist down—only the torso.
Martial artists can do the drill from the horse stance.

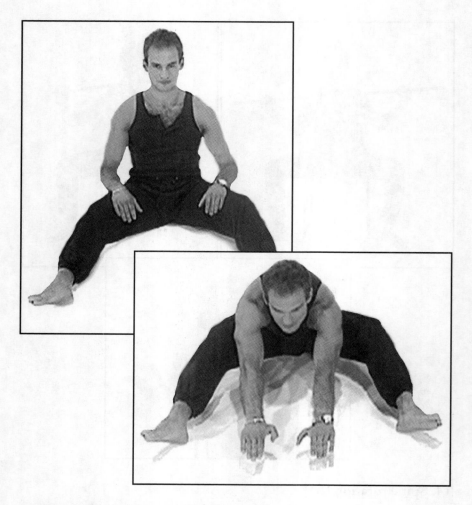

15. Forward spine flexion [MF]

Sit on the floor with your feet comfortably wide and your knees slightly bent to make sure your hamstrings do not interfere with this mostly back exercise.

Smoothly reach forward touching the floor in front of you with your hands. Try to reach further and further.

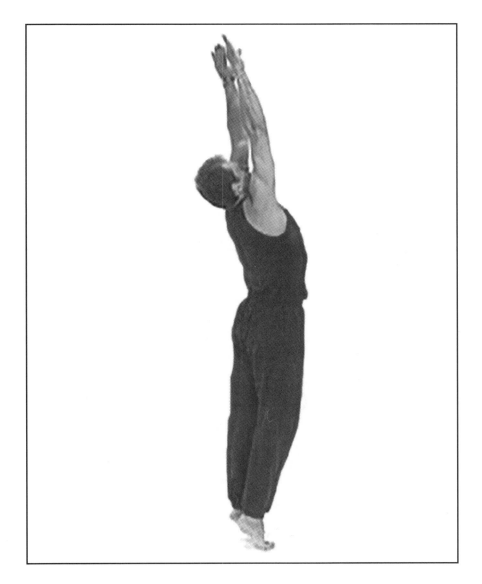

16. Spine extension [M]

Inhale as deep as you can, coming up on your toes and "growing" to reach the ceiling.

Exhale as you relax and come down.

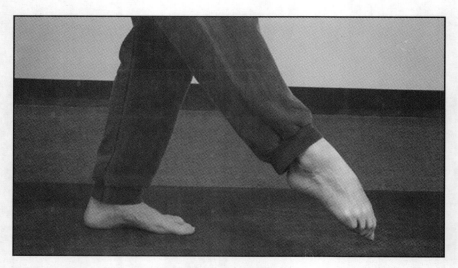

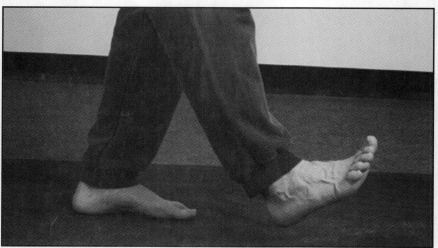

17. Toe fist [MF]

Do the same thing you have done with your hands. Curl you toes in a "fist," simultaneously extending—pointing—your foot. Then pull them back—toes towards your nose! —and flex your foot the same way.

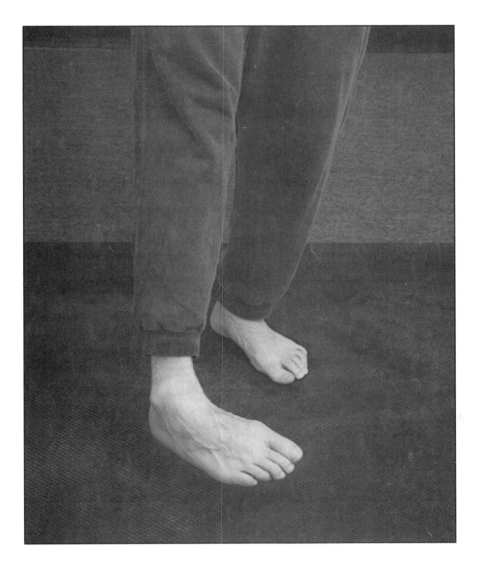

18. Ankle rotation [M]

Make circles with your feet. That's all!

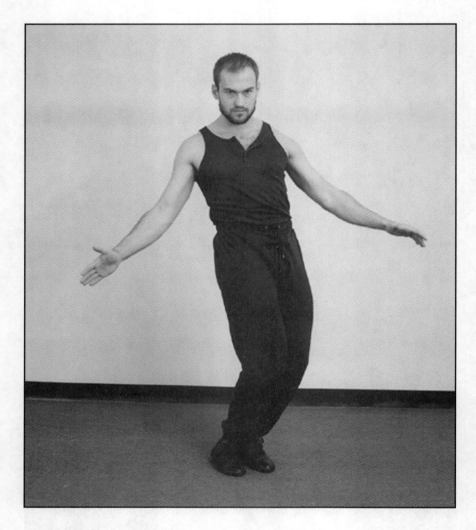

19. Knee circles [M]

Keep your knees together and make small circles.
I repeat—small. The knees' natural lateral range of motion
is only a couple of degrees and trying to force out more
could stretch the ligaments and weaken your knees.

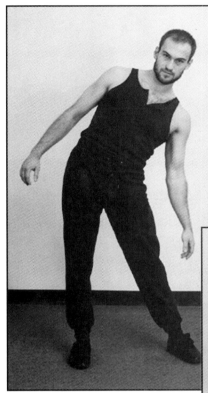

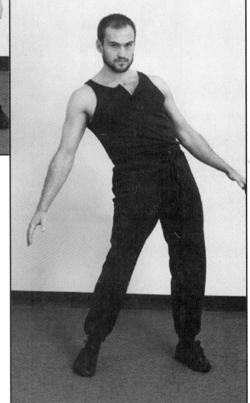

20. Hoola hoop [M]

Keep your feet shoulder wide and make circles with your hips, while keeping your shoulders stationary. Gradually increase the amplitude.

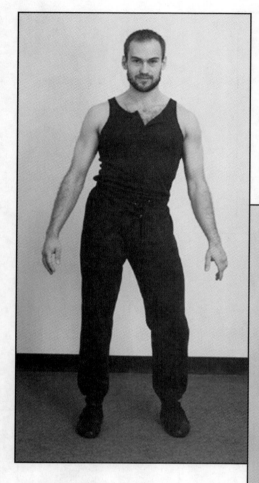

21. Belly dancing [M]

I learned this drill from Vladimir Zadiran, a former USSR karate champion. You would have died laughing—literally—watching his toughs belly dancing at the KGB Dynamo Sports Club dojo.

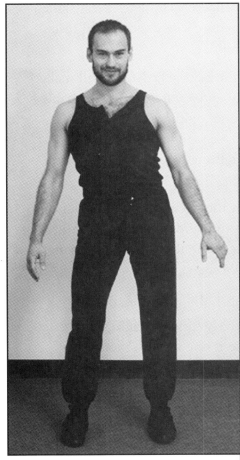

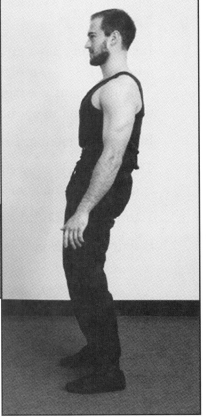

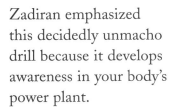

Zadiran emphasized
this decidedly unmacho
drill because it develops
awareness in your body's
power plant.

No matter what sport you play, most of your power should
come from the hip. Even in boxing, considered by many
an arm sport, only 20% of the punch is the arm and
shoulder, the hips and torso rotation are responsible for
80% of the force!

These numbers apply to elite level athletes. Less skilled people tend to use more arm. Belly dancing will teach them to emphasize the hips.

Belly dancing is a must for martial artists. It will make your kicks more powerful and accurate and will enable you to change one kick into another easily and with no telegraphing. If you have seen world kickboxing champion Bill Wallace fighting, you will know what I mean.

Belly dancing has a great therapeutic effect on your hip joints. It helps your digestion and regularity as well. The movement massages the inner organs, improving the circulation in a usually stagnant area.

But enough talking. Let's do it.

Tilt your pelvis consecutively forward, right, back, and left. Eventually make it one smooth motion.

Your knees will bend slightly. It is OK.

Practice this exercise at home—alone!

22. Squats [M]

Squats are excellent for the hip and knee joints,
but you must do them right.

Keep your heels on the floor and your weight
on your heels.

Keep your shins nearly vertical. Don't let your knees
move forward even in the bottom position. You should
be able to do this exercise wearing stiff ski boots!

Your knees should point in the same direction as your
feet—forward, or slightly out. Don't let them buckle in.

Sit back, rather than down.

If you squat correctly, your center of gravity will be behind
your feet and you will hold on to something for balance.
A doorway works well.

Hold on to the doorway at your waist level, no higher.
Stand almost inside the door.

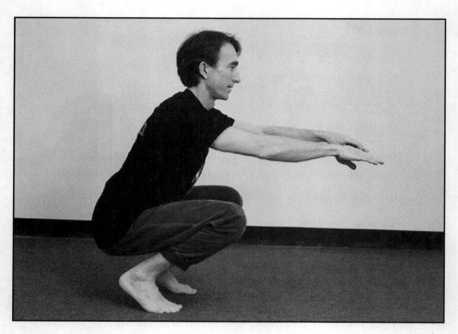

Wrong way to do squats

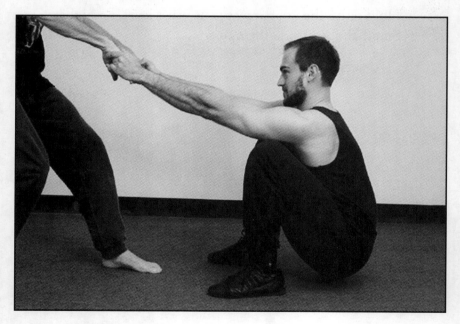

Correct way to do squats.

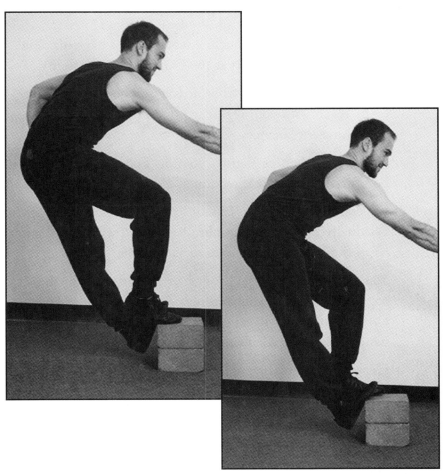

23. Stair calf stretch [F]

For a great calf stretch you need a stair step, or something similar.

Stand on the edge of the step with the balls of your feet.
Hold on to the railing for balance.
Lean back, shifting most of your weight on one foot
and stretching your calf.

Switch, as if walking. Gradually increase the depth.

24. Front hand kick *(hamstrings)* [F]

This Soviet commando drill enables you to have maximal speed in your kicks even at the limit of your flexibility.

Hold your hand out in front of you at a height you can easily reach with your leg. It is OK to hold on to something for balance.

Keep your other leg slightly bent, its knee and foot pointing in the same direction at a forty five degree angle.

Kick your hand with a straight leg. Start slow and low. Gradually increase the amplitude, leading with your hand. Keep the kicking leg as relaxed as possible.

You are not going to feel your hamstrings much in the beginning, because your hip flexor muscles, whose job is to raise your leg, will fatigue quickly. Relax between reps, switch your legs when tired, and be patient.

Hit your hand with your shin—not the other way around. Don't hold your hand too high! There should be no doubt in your mind that you can reach it without injuring yourself.

Stop increasing the stretch when you feel that your hamstring is going to tighten up if you go any higher—not when it does! Once again, a properly performed dynamic stretch is terminated right before the stretch reflex fires!

Vary the plane of movement: move your hand around, switch hands.

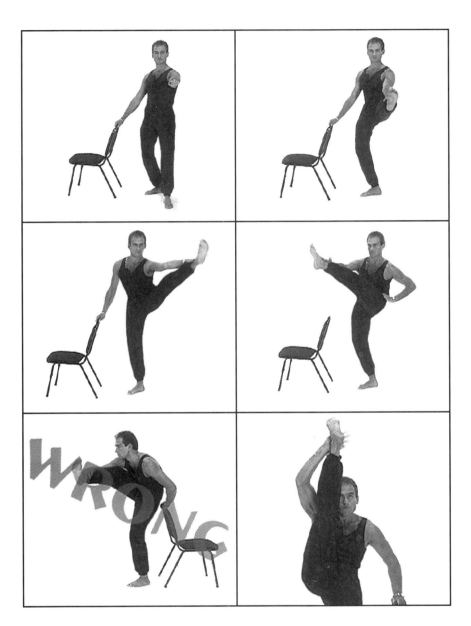

Front hand kick *(hamstrings)* **[F]**

25. Side hand kick *(inner thighs: hip adductors)* [F]

This drill is tough to master. Pay attention.

Hold on to something for balance. Arrange your kicking leg, torso, and your planted foot in one plane. The position is similar to the taekwondo side kick.

Thrust your hips forward, rotate your toes slightly down, and pull them back at the same time.

Without these fine points the stretch will not work. If you simply try to raise your leg to the side—your femur will jam into your pelvis. No go!

Kick your hand, as in the front kick.

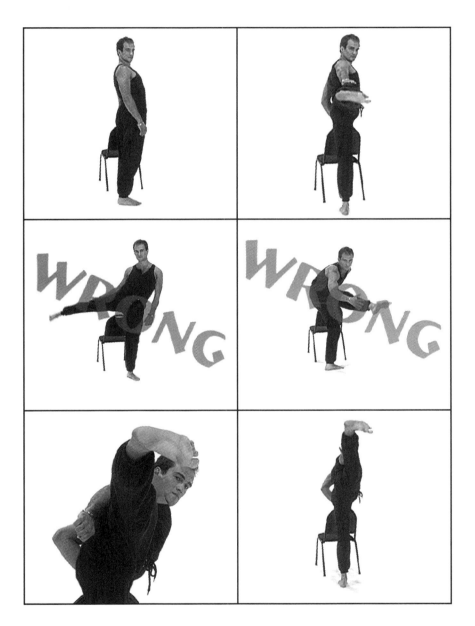

Side hand kick *(inner thighs: hip adductors)* **[F]**

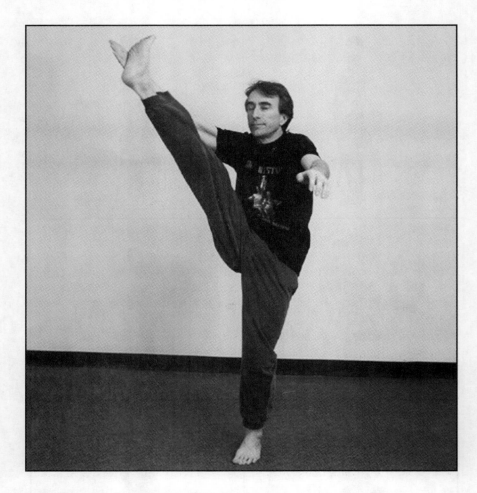

26. Outside crescent hand kick *(inner thighs: internal hip rotators)* [F]

Stretch your arm out to the side with your palm facing forward.

Swing your leg on the same side of the body in a circular motion towards your hand. Kick your hand with the outside of your foot.

Beginners should hit their hand with their knee, rather then the foot.

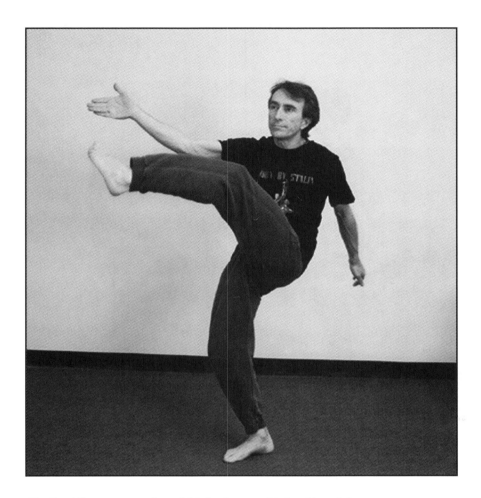

27. Inside crescent hand kick *(outer thighs: hip abductors, external hip rotators)* [F]

Stretch your arm out to the side with your palm facing forward.

Swing your leg on the opposite side of the body in a circular motion towards your hand. Kick your hand with the inside of your foot.

Beginners should hit their hand with their knee, rather then the foot.

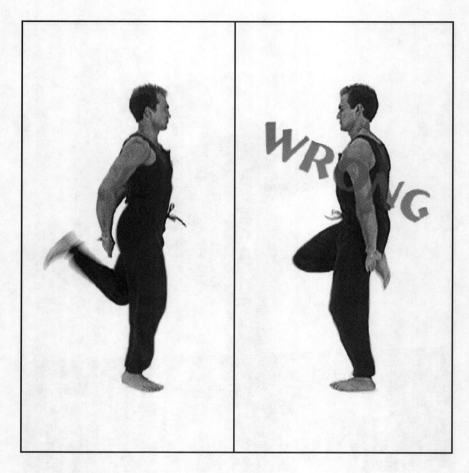

28. Butt kicks *(quads)* [F]

Put your hands behind your butt and kick them.

Your knees must not move forward. You should be able to do this stretch facing the wall!

When you become proficient, try this exercise while running.

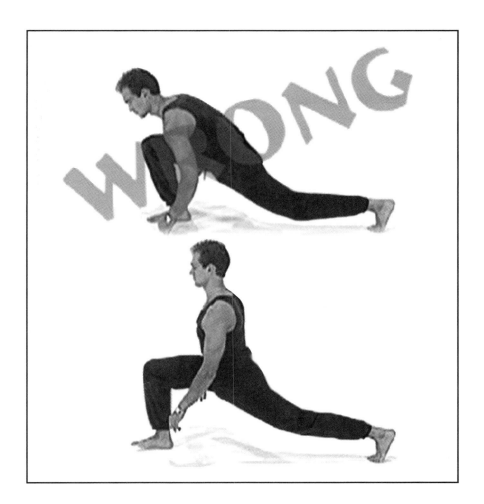

29. Lunge *(hip flexors)* [F]

Keep your torso and the rear leg straight.

Keep your front shin vertical and don't let your knee hang over your foot.

Float up and down.

It is OK to hold on to something for balance. It is not OK to lean on your thigh.

Isometric and Extreme Range Stretches

Make sure to carefully study the fine points of pneumomuscular and isometric stretching in Part II before doing the following exercises!

The stretches below can be done in either PFT, or STI format.

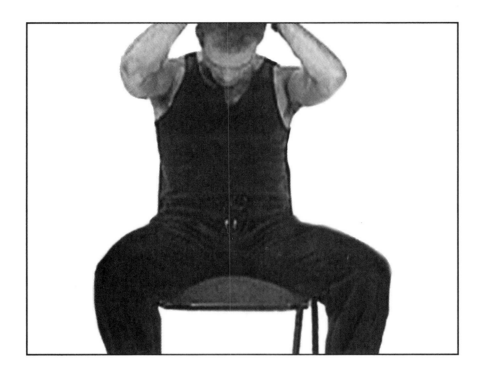

30. Neck forward flexion

Not everybody needs more flexible necks—if you can touch your chest with your chin, how much further can you go?—yet many people should do neck isometrics.

Isometric stretches are great for relieving the tension in your neck, regardless of its source—getting tired, or getting fired.

There is no point in stretching the front of your neck: it is not safe and nobody carries stress there anyway.

So we'll work on the back of your neck.

Clasp your hands behind your neck and tuck your chin in. Push with your head against your hands. Relax. Increase the stretch, if possible. Repeat.

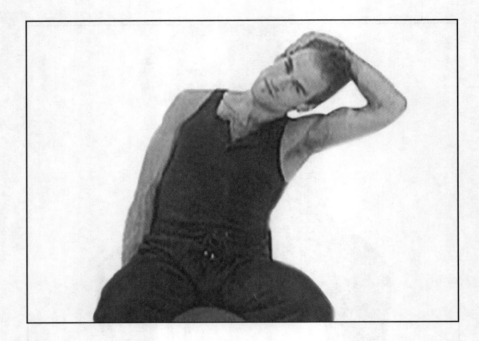

31. Neck lateral flexion

To stretch the side of your neck sit in a chair and grab its base with one hand. Tilt your head in the opposite direction.

Push your head against your hand, gradually increasing the pressure.

Relax.

32. Neck rotation *(not illustrated)*

Make sure you keep your head upright throughout the stretch. No twisting—it is not a ninja movie!

Place you hand on the side of your head, and push.

Push—relax—increase the stretch. Same drill.

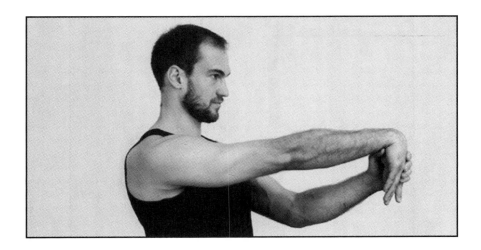

33. Wrist flexion

Straighten out your arm in front of you with your wrist bent.

Try to straighten out your wrist against your other hand.

Relax. Increase the stretch.

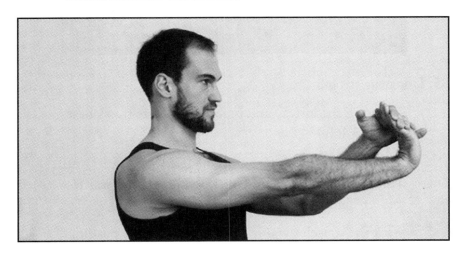

34. Wrist extension

Do everything the same as in the last drill, except bend your wrist in the opposite direction.

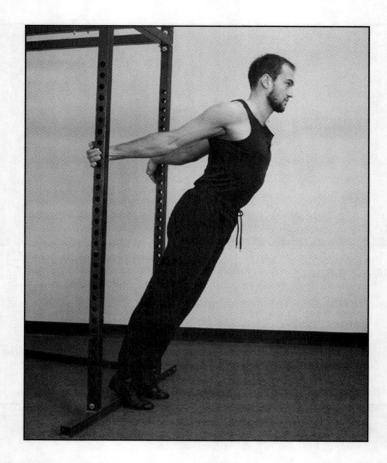

35. Doorway stretch

Stand in a doorway and grab the sides at your chest or waist level.

Keeping your elbows slightly bent, lean forward until your shoulders tighten. Don't bend from the waist, rather "fall" forward.

Flex the muscles you have just stretched by pushing against the doorway.

Suddenly relax and drop forward a little, increasing the stretch.

Hold the last contraction for up to 30 seconds.

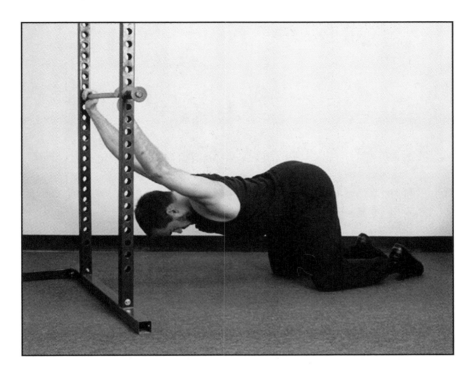

36. Table top lat stretch

Kneel in front of a table, or stand in front of a refrigerator, and put your hands on top of it, shoulder wide.

Push down, then relax and drop.

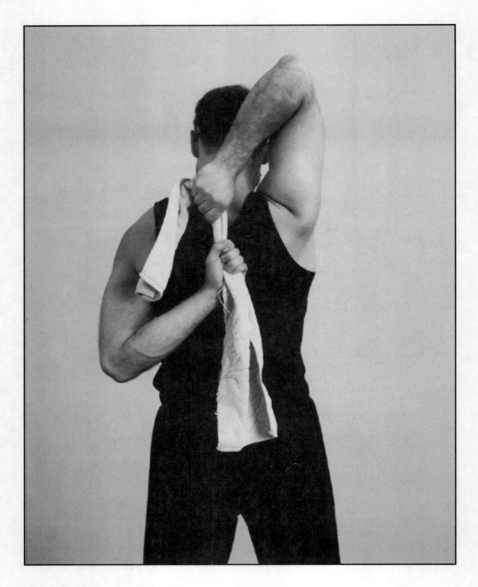

37. Archer stretch *(lats and triceps)*

Hold a towel behind your back as shown.

Try to tear the towel apart.

Relax, and move your hands closer together, "climbing" the towel.

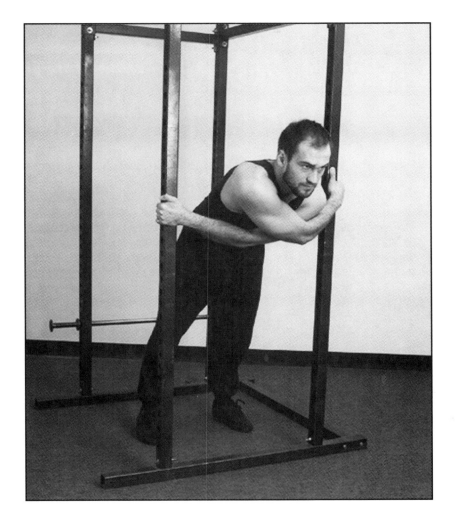

38. Crossover stretch *(upper back, midback & back of the shoulders)*

Cross your arms and grab the doorway as shown.

Lean forward. You should feel a stretch in your upper back, between your shoulder blades, and in the back of your shoulders.

Pull on the doorway, trying to "uncross" your arms

Relax, drop, repeat.

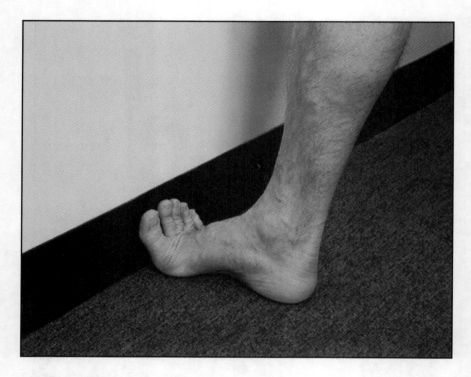

39. Toe extension

This is a martial arts stretch. It helps to keep your toes pulled back when you kick with the ball of your foot.

Sit on a chair facing a wall. Keep your feet on the floor, your toes touching the wall. Don't wear shoes.

Push with your toes against the wall, trying to straighten them out.

Relax and move your feet closer to the wall, as your toes curl back.

40. Standing calf stretch *(gastrocnemius)*—not illustrated

For this stretch you might need extra weight, a dumbbell, or a suitcase, because the calf muscles have very good leverage. You also can use various calf strength training machines, or a leg press machine.

Stand on the edge of a stair step on the ball of one foot. Hold a dumbbell in your hand on the same side. Hold on to the railing for balance with the other hand.

Lean back and let your heel sink, stretching your calf muscle.

Flex your calf.

Release and increase the depth.

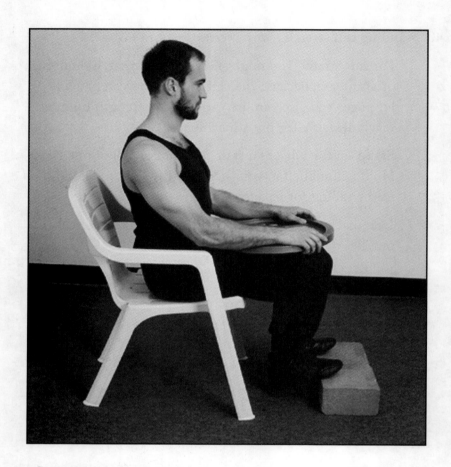

41. Seated calf stretch *(soleus)*

This drill is useful if your sport requires high levels of ankle flexibility when your knees are bent. Shotokan karate is an example.

Use a health club seated calf machine, if possible. If not, improvise:

Sit in a chair with a weight in your lap, your kid or spouse will do!

Place the balls of your feet on top of a solid block and let your heels sink.

Flex your calves. Release and increase the depth.

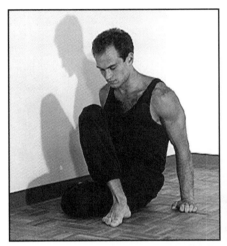 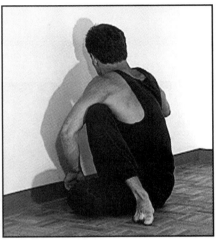

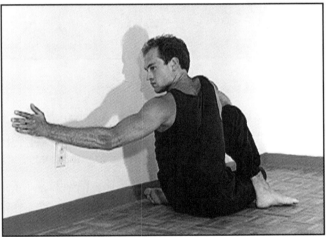

42. "Pretzel" *(spine rotation & outer thighs: hip abductors)*

Sit by a wall with one leg folded underneath you. Keep your back perfectly straight and your chest out.

Apply pressure to your knee with your other elbow. At the same time push your hand against the wall.

Relax, rotate your truck while sliding your hand on the wall.

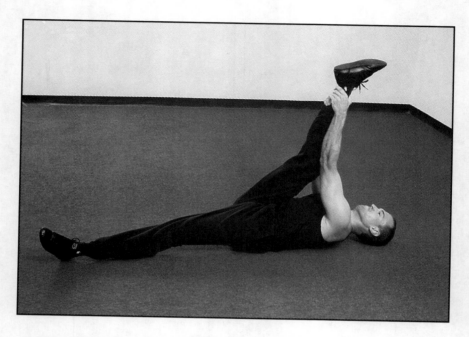

43. Hamstring towel stretch

Lie on your back with a towel in your hands. The towel should wrap around the instep of one leg. Keep your hands high on the towel so your arms are nearly straight.

Raise a straight leg, the one with the towel, as far as you can. Keep the other leg straight and on the floor. The foot of the leg you are stretching can be either pointed or flexed towards you. In the latter case your calf will get stretched as well.

Inhale and tighten up your entire body while pushing with your foot against the towel.

Release the air with the tension and immediately—but not fast!—pull on the towel toward you to increase the stretch.

Do it in small increments, an inch or less. Move your hands up the towel whenever you can; it will make your arms' job easier and will allow you to focus on your hamstring.

Throughout the stretch make sure your butt or the other leg do not come off the floor. Pushing your chest high and arching your back will help.

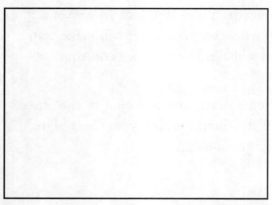

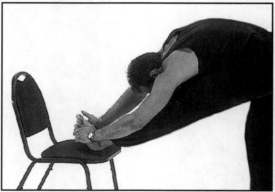

44. Hamstring chair stretch

Stand in front of a chair with one foot on top of it, its toes pointing up. Keep the knee of the other leg pointing in the same direction as its foot, forward, or slightly out. Don't let your knee buckle in.

Lean forward, putting as much weight on your stretched hamstring as possible. It is OK to round your back, unless you are super flexible. It is OK to hold on to something for balance, as long as you do not put your weight on your hands.

Push down into the bench with your heel.

Release and let yourself drop forward.

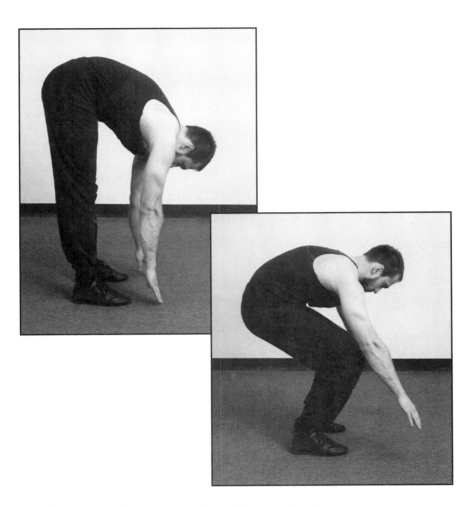

45. Toe touch *(hamstrings, glutes & lower back)*

Stand a foot away from a wall, facing away from it.
Keep your feet a comfortable distance apart and your
weight on your heels. The wall is there to catch you
if you overbalance. Slowly bend over until you reach
a comfortable stretch. There is no need to keep your
back straight, unless you are already very flexible in
your hamstrings.

Let your arms hang loose or fold them on your chest.

Inhale as deep as possible and tighten every muscle in your body, while digging your heels hard into the floor. Hold your breath and tension for a few seconds, then suddenly let all the air go with the tension. You will drop and fold forward, thanks to the weight of your torso.

Relax for a moment, then inhale and tighten again and repeat. When you tighten, make sure that you stay down and do not decrease the stretch by straightening out your back

When you have reached your limit for the day, bend your knees first—it is essential for your back health!—and only then straighten out.

46. Powerlifter's back and hamstring stretch—*not illustrated*

I have modified one of powerlifting guru Louie Simmons' exercises into a very effective stretch. Sit on the floor with your legs straight. Hold a barbell low on your back. If you keep it high, the bar will roll down on your neck later in the stretch. The bar should be very light: 10% of your squat or deadlift at most. In the relaxed phase of this stretch the load will supported by the lower back ligaments. A heavy weight could stretch them which would weaken your back.

Inhale as deep as possible and tighten every muscle in your body, while digging your heels hard into the floor. Hold your breath and tension for a few seconds, then suddenly let all the air go with the tension. You will drop and fold forward, thanks to the weight on your shoulders.

You do not need to keep your back flat or arched unless you are already very flexible. Keep your toes pointed up. If they just fall out when you relax, have a training partner hold them in place, or wedge them in somewhere. Inhale and tighten again and repeat. When you tighten, make sure that you stay down and do not decrease the stretch by lifting the bar.

47. Spine decompression

An acquaintance of mine, the chief detective of a police department in one of the former Soviet republics, was self conscious about his height—or rather lack of it—and took up to daily hanging from a pull up bar. His taller wife would wrap her arms and legs around his waist and hang on to him to provide extra resistance.

The strange exercise paid off—the fellow gained over an inch in height after awhile.

Sandwiched between the vertebrae, your spinal disks act as shock absorbers.

They hold water like sponges to do their job. Unfortunately, the never relenting gravity keeps squeezing the moisture out of them. The disks eventually dry out, get thin and brittle. As a result, your spine shrinks, stiffens up, and becomes more injury prone.

When astronauts return to earth they are a couple of inches taller then before the space flight, thanks to zero G. If NASA is not hiring, decompressing the spine by hanging on a pull up bar, head up, or upside down as it was the rage twenty years ago, will let the disks to absorb more moisture. It will not only help you to reclaim your youthful height, but will do a lot for your spinal health and mobility.

When you apply the pneumomuscular stretching breathing pattern to the overhead bar hang, you will be blown away with how much better your back feels after the drill!

Hang from a pull up bar. Inhale as deep as possible and tighten every muscle in your body, making sure that you do not pull up higher.

Hold your breath and tension for a few seconds, then suddenly let all the air go with the tension. You will drop, sort of "getting taller."

Repeat. Alternate the palms forward and palms back grips every workout.

Ideally, you should do this stretch every day, many times throughout the day.

Still, twice a week is better than nothing.

Make sure to hang out after lifting weights. Also, the spine extension stretch, the hip flexor stretch, and the splits will go a lot smoother if you precede them with spinal decompression.

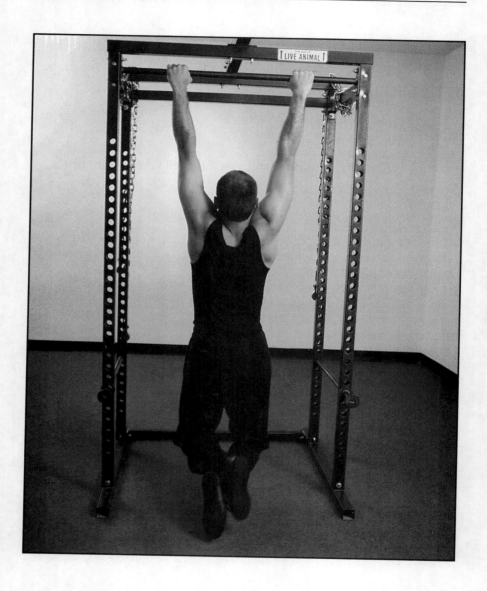

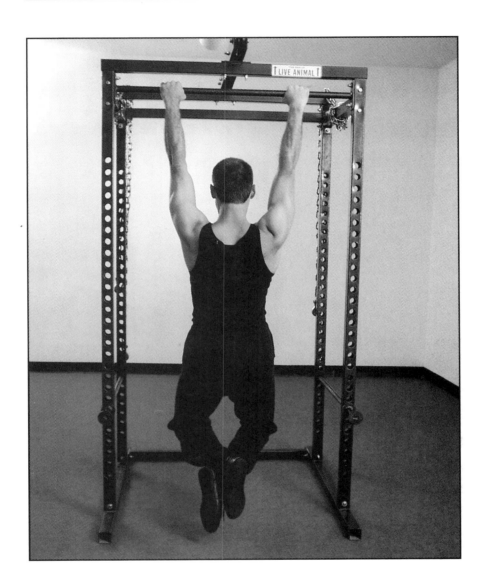

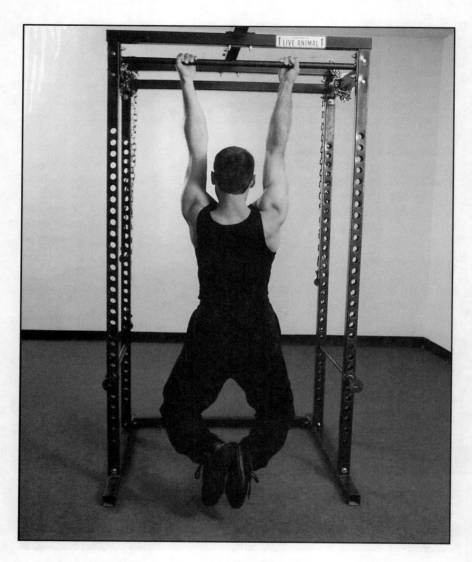

Spine decompression with a different grip.

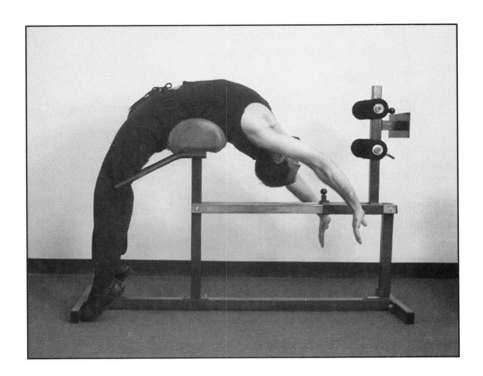

48. Spine extension

The conventional back extension stretches, the "bridge" and the "cobra," jam the spine in one spot—where it hurts—and often cause damage to the disks and facet joints.

The new stretch is much safer because it opens up the vertebrae to allow more room for the disks.

You need a curved padded surface to distribute the stress evenly throughout the spine, rather than jam it in one spot.

Standing with your back towards the pad inhale deeply and "grow," separating the vertebrae to allow your disks more room to play with.

Still holding your breath, lean back trying to "wrap" your back around the pad.

Flex your abs.

Relax and drop down an inch or so, at the same time trying to "elongate" your spine.

If you experience pain in in your back, you are doing the stretch wrong.

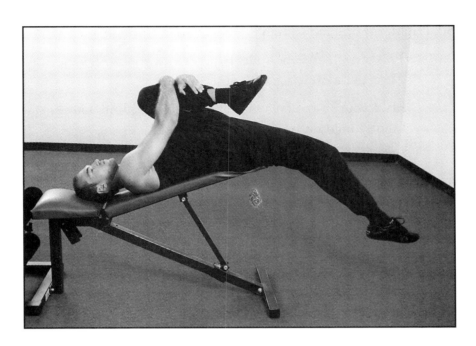

49. Low back stress hip flexor stretch

Lie on your back on the edge of a tall table. Bring one knee toward your chest and hold it there throughout the stretch. Let the other leg hang off the edge.

Inhale and tighten your body, especially the top of the thigh of the hanging leg.

Release the tension with your breath and let the leg drop a little. Eventually wear an ankle weight. Your Rollerblades will do!

50. Hip flexor & quad stretch

This stretch and the splits hyperextend your spine. Clear these exercises with your doctor.

Place your instep on a tall table or chair behind you. Lightly hold on to something for balance.

Lean back and push down on the table with your instep, as if you are trying to kick. Keep your hips squared throughout the stretch.

Relax your thigh suddenly. Your hip will drop a little. Don't lean forward!

Now extend your hip back as far as possible. Imagine making your leg longer, or pulling your hip out of its socket.

You can also stretch your hip flexors with your knee on the floor. Make sure to use adequate padding for your patella.

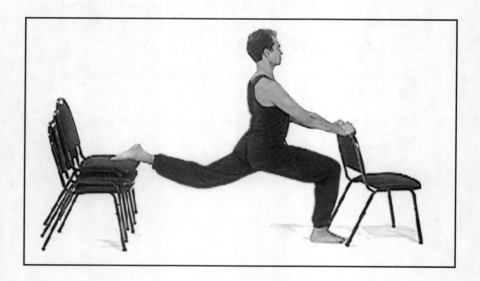

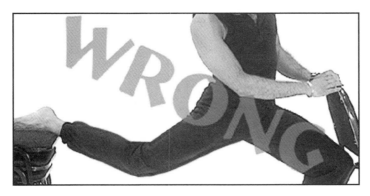

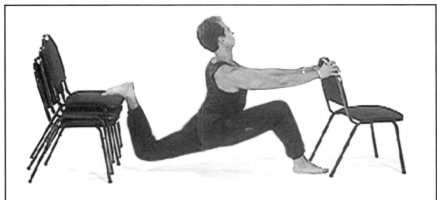

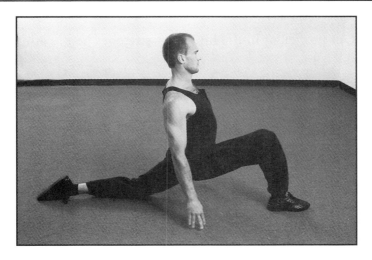

Hip flexor and quad stretch *(floor version)*

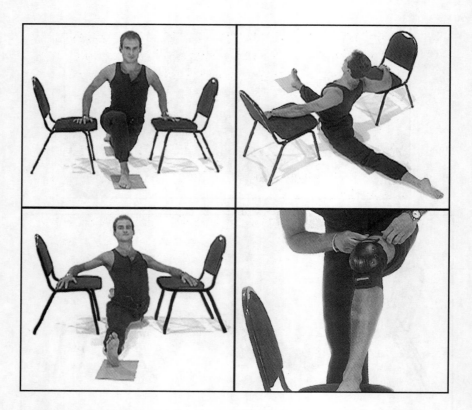

51. Front split

Get proficient in the hip flexor stretches before attempting the split.

Do the split on the carpet. Put a newspaper, or a folded under your front heel and rear knee to slide easier. Your rear knee will need some padding: a roller skating knee pad, or a folded towel.

Surround yourself with two chairs to spot you in case you lose balance. Barely touch the chairs. Don't lean on them unless you are falling!

Lean back, keeping your hips squared. Squeezing your butt will help with the alignment and balance. Pinch the floor with your front heel and rear knee, as if you are trying to slide up.

Relax suddenly, and let yourself slide deeper into the split. Don't lean forward.

Support yourself on your arms and extend your rear hip like in the previous stretch.

Hold the last tension for 30 seconds. Scream your heart out!

52. Hip flexor, glute and outer thigh stretch

Get down on one knee—use some padding—with your front leg folded underneath your. Play with your position to make sure you are not wrenching your front knee.

Keep your hips squared off—squeezing your butt will help—and your torso upright. Hold on to something for balance if you wish.

Inhale and tighten, then exhale and relax. Your hip will drop lower and you will feel the stretch in your front glute and abductor.

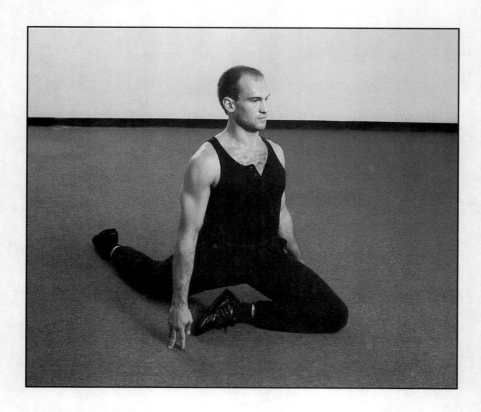

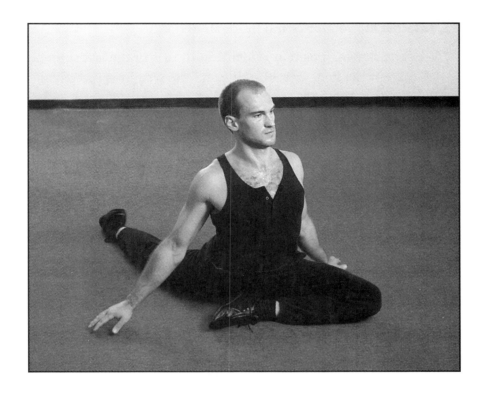

53. Internal hip rotator & hip flexor stretch

The starting position is identical to that of the last stretch, except the knee is a 90° angle and the weight is placed on your ankle, rather than the knee.

Inhale and flex. When the tension is released, you will sink down and the front hip will externally rotate around the axis shown on the picture.

Make sure to assume a position that does not wrench your knee and hip. If you can't—ditch this horrible stretch!

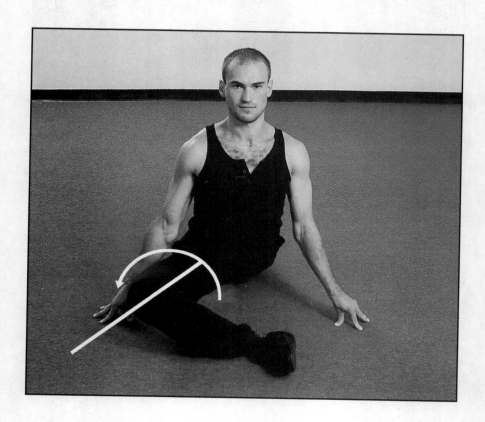

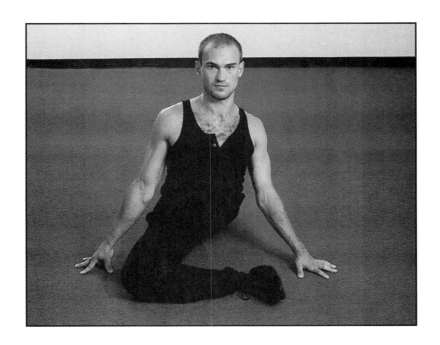

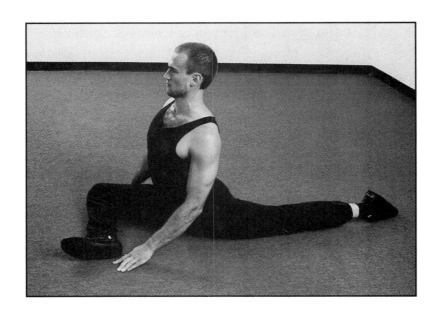

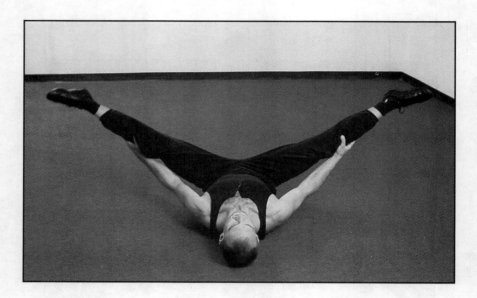

54. Groin stretch #1

Lie on your back with your legs pointing straight up, your knees locked. Place your hands under your thighs, close to the back sides of your knees, to make sure that your legs do not drop down and remain at a ninety degree angle to your torso. Holding on to your pants is an option.

Spread your legs as far as comfortably possible. Now inhale maximally and tighten every muscle in your body, especially your hip adductors, or inner thighs.

Hold your breath and tension for a few seconds, then suddenly let all the air go with the tension. Your legs will spread further. Don't let them drop far, an inch per tension/release cycle will do. Don't pull down with your hands, they are only for helping you do keep your legs in the right place.

Now arch your back while inhaling and pushing your chest out. At the same time point your toes and sort of

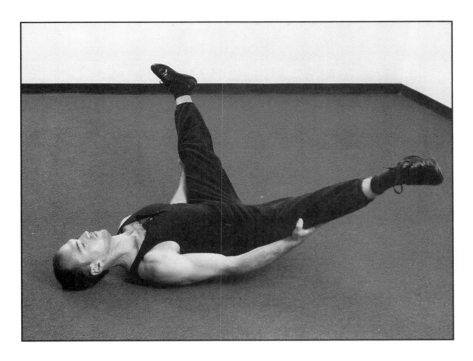

"make your legs longer." Imagine that you are pulling your hips out of their sockets. You will find that this maneuver will significantly increase your range of motion. Feel free to use this trick in sports, martial, arts, or dance techniques.

Alternate tension/release cycles with arching your back and "growing" your legs.

It is OK to pull down gently with your arms when you are approaching your current limit. And make sure to use your arms to keep your legs at a ninety degree angle to your torso.

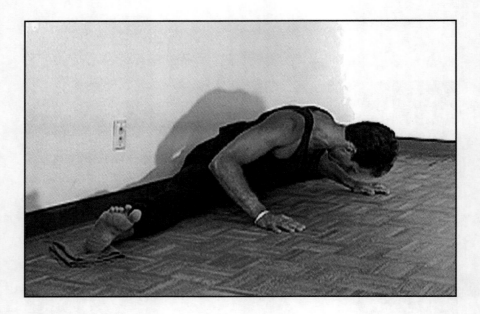

55. Groin stretch #2

Sit on the floor and spread your legs wide.

Without touching the floor, slowly lean forward until your inner thighs tighten up.

Flex your groin muscles even more, then relax an let yourself drop forward. Keep the weight on your adductors and use your hands only for spotting.

When you can go no further, sit up and spread your legs wider.

Repeat the sequence.

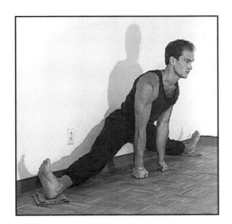
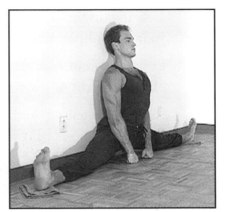

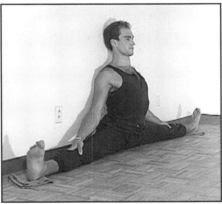

56. Wall split

This is a more extreme version of the previous stretch. You can combine both in one set, if you wish.

Sit on the floor with your back to the wall and spread your legs. Slide newspapers under your feet if you exercise on a carpet. On the photo I use folded towels on a hardwood floor.

Set a chair or a step stool in front of you for additional safety. I don't in the photo because it would have blocked your view of the stretch. A ballet bar above you works even better.

Leaning on the step stool, lift your hips and spread your legs a little. Keep your toes pointing up.

Pinch the floor, as if trying to slide up. Keep most of your weight on your heels.

Release the tension and drop an inch or so. Let your feet slide out—not forward.

Lean back against the wall when you are low enough. Arch your back and force your chest out. Continue the tense/drop sequence.

When you have reached the floor, start over— lift yourself up and spread your legs a little further.

57. (Suspended) side split

Here it comes—the "wishbone!" It is as painful as it looks.

Clear this drill with your doctor if you have knee problems.

Before you attempt a side split, you have to understand its mechanics. You cannot do it by simply spreading your legs out to the sides—your femurs will jam into the pelvis.

You have to either externally rotate your hips and point your toes up, as in the wall split, or arch your back and thrust your hips forward, as far as your heels.

Also, "pull your hips out of their sockets making your legs longer."

First, do the wall split. For safety arrange three chairs around you: two over your legs, and one in the front. They are not shown on the picture to give you a better view.

If you are flexible enough to try suspended splits, instead of newspapers use phone books inside sturdy manila envelopes. I am not a big fan of suspended splits between chairs, a la Van Damme. If you fall—you will be out of commission for good.

Place your hands slightly behind you on the side chairs. Lift your hips and push them forward until they are level with your heels. At the same time turn your toes forward. Don't lean forward!

Carefully transfer the weight from your hand to your legs. Still touch the chairs lightly and be ready to catch yourself if necessary.

Pinch the floor with your feet as if trying to slide them together.

Release and slide out. Imagine making your legs longer. It is OK to lean on your arms and rest in this position for awhile.

Shift your weight back to your legs and repeat.

Hold the last contraction for 30 seconds, or do the following dynamic strength exercise.

Shift enough weight on your hands to enable you to slide up from the split—although with difficulty—using your groin muscles. Go up a couple of inches, then all the way down.

Here is another way to get down in a side split.

Stand on two magazine covers holding on to a solid object, a ballet bar, for example. It is there to spot you in case of trouble, not to support you throughout the stretch! Your feet should be turned slightly out.

Inhale, tighten up, then release the tension and slide out an inch or so.

Throughout the stretch keep your hips level with your feet, not behind, and your torso upright. You will never do a split if your butt shoots back!

Release and slide out.

Push the walls apart! Remember, just spreading your legs does not cut it!

Shift your weight back to your legs, and repeat.

If you hit a plateau, remember, it is all in your head!
A suspended side split, like a fire walk, is an act of faith.
It is not psychobabble, but a fact. The centers in your
brain which govern the muscular length and tension
and your emotions are intimately connected. No wonder
Indian Yogi use flexibility as a litmus test of the state
of the practitioner's mind! If you do not believe that
you can do a wishbone—you won't. And the other way
around. Have faith. It can be done!

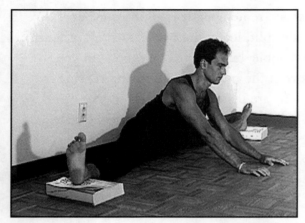

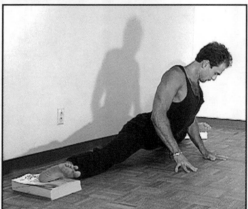

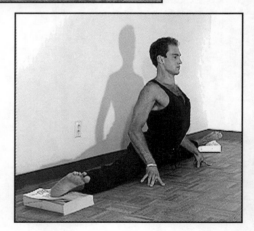

(Suspended) side split

Stretches with Weights

58. Stiff-legged deadlift

This is an excellent drill for improving your hamstring flexibility and extreme range strength.

Shift your weight on your heels and keep it there throughout the set. Inhale deeply, arching your back and looking up.

Maintaining a tight arch in your back and holding your breath, push your glutes back, letting the barbell descend close to your shins.

Go as deep as you can while keeping your back flat. Hinge only in the hip joint, there should be no movement of the spine.

Lift the weight by driving your hips through. Stand straight, without leaning back. Exhale.

Doing the stiff-legged deadlift with your toes on a platform has the added benefit of increasing your calf flexibility.

Wrong

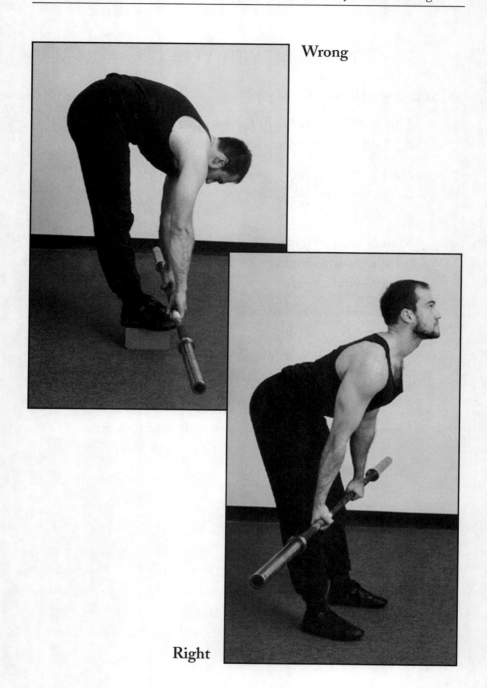

Right

Stiff-legged deadlift *(right & wrong)*

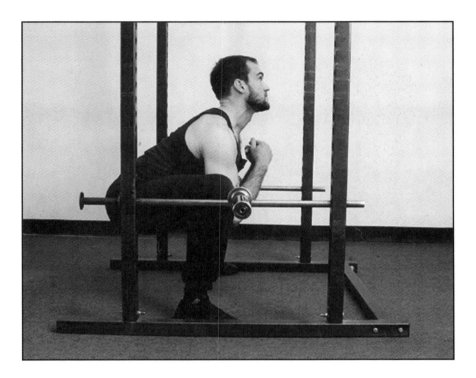

59. Spider lift

Start in a power rack, with the barbell slightly below your knees and your feet slightly wider than your shoulders. As you become more advanced, you will lower the bar, eventually to the floor, and set your feet wider.

Stand with your shins touching the bar. Point your toes out at a natural to you angle. The wider and lower you go, the more turnout you will need. It is imperative that your knees always point in the same direction as your toes! Allowing your knees to buckle in will make the exercise less effective and could cause damage to your knee and hip joints.

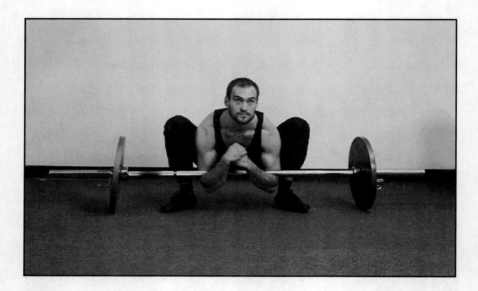

Sit back—not down—keeping your shins vertical and pushing your knees out. You might need to hold on to the power rack to keep your balance as you are getting into the starting position.

Place the bar in the crooks of your elbows as shown. It is OK to use padding. Make sure that your hips are below your knees, your weight is on your heels, and your shoulders are directly above the bar—not in front of it.

Inhale as deeply as possible in this constricted position and look up. At the same time arch, or at least flatten your back. Do not let your butt tuck in.

Push the floor away while pushing your knees out at the same time. Don't let your hips rise too soon. Keep looking up and stay as upright as you can. Don't let your knees move forward. Imagine that you are stuck in cement up to your knees.

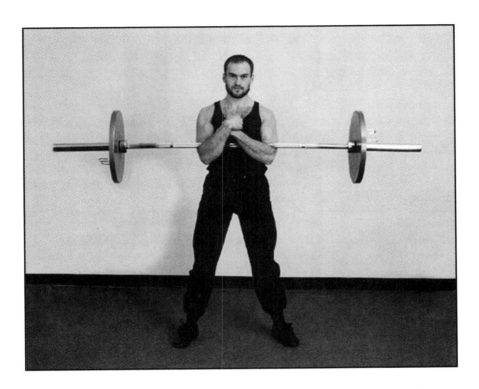

Exhale as you reach the top. Inhale again, and sit back (don't bend over!). When the bar reaches the bottom position, it should be in front of your knees—not on top of them. Your shins must remain vertical.

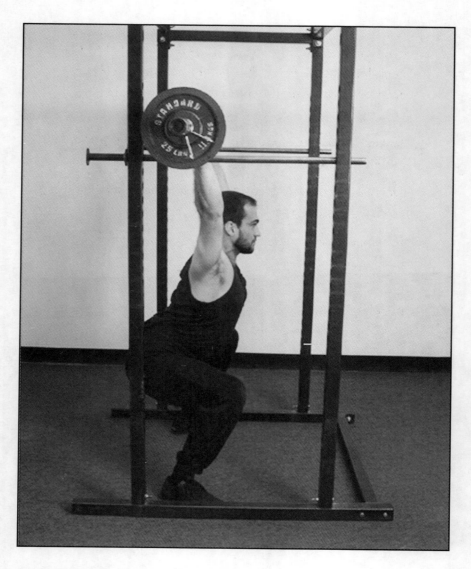

60. Overhead squat

I designed this exercise specifically for improving the hip flexibility in the squat. After I showed it to 900-pound-squatter Dr. Fred Clary, many lifters from the Twin Cities Gym in St. Paul, Minnesota, picked up on it.

Do the exercise in a power rack. Hold a light barbell over your head in the position for the press behind the neck lockout. Keeping the weight overhead is what enforces proper alignment and makes the exercise so effective.

If your shoulders lack flexibility, develop it with the table top lat stretch.

Don't lean back. You should look like you have just landed from a jump.

Inhale, and sit back on your heels, pushing your butt back and knees out.

Go as deep as you can, as long as your knees do not buckle in or move excessively forward and the barbell stays behind your neck.

Hold that position, breathing shallow, until you collapse. When you do, fall back, still pushing your knees out. Hold on to the bar—it will catch you when it hits the safety pin.

The safety pin in the power rack must be set an inch or two below the point of collapse!

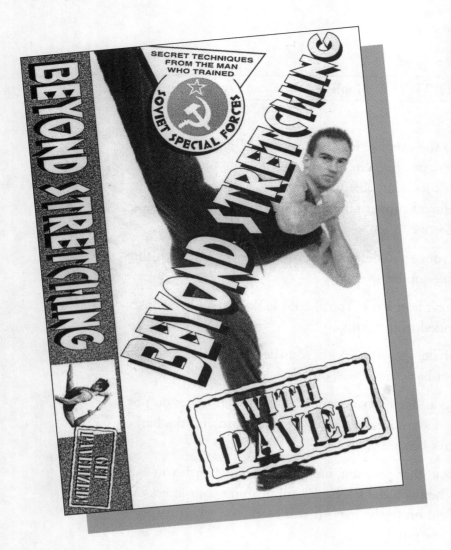

Order the companion video,
BEYOND STRETCHING.
Now, for only $29.^{95}

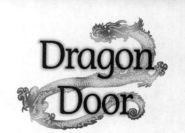

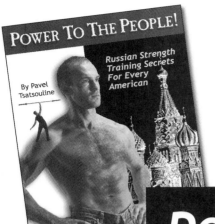

POWER TO THE PEOPLE!

RUSSIAN STRENGTH TRAINING SECRETS FOR EVERY AMERICAN

By Pavel Tsatsouline

8½" x 11" 124 pages, over 100 photographs and illustrations—$34.95 #B10

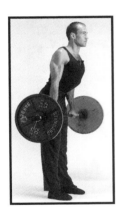

How would you like to own a world class body—<u>whatever your present condition</u>— by doing only two exercises, for twenty minutes a day?" A body so lean, ripped and powerful looking, you won't believe your own reflection when you catch yourself in the mirror.

And what if you could do it without a single supplement, without having to waste your time at a gym and with only a 150 bucks of simple equipment?

And how about not only being stronger than you've ever been in your life, but having higher energy and better performance in whatever you do?

How would you like to have an instant download of the world's <u>absolutely most effective strength secrets?</u> To possess exactly the same knowledge that created world-champion athletes—and the strongest bodies of their generation?"

Pavel Tsatsouline's *Power to the People!— Russian Strength Training Secrets for Every American* delivers all of this and more.

As **Senior Science Editor for Joe Weider's** *Flex* magazine, **Jim Wright** is recognized as one of the world's premier authorities on strength training. Here's more of what he had to say:

"Whether you're young or old, a beginner or an elite athlete, training in your room or in the most high tech facility, if there was only one book I could recommend to help you reach your ultimate physical potential, this would be it.

Simple, concise and truly reader friendly, this amazing book contains it all—everything you need to know—what exercises (only two!), how to do them (unique detailed information you'll find nowhere else), and why.

Follow its advice and, believe it or not, you'll be stronger and more injury-resistant immediately. I guarantee it. I only wish I'd had a book like this when I first began training.

Follow this program for three months and you'll not only be amazed but hooked. It is the ultimate program for "Everyman" AND Woman! I thought I knew a lot with a Ph.D. and 40 years of training experience...but I learned a lot and it's improved my training significantly."

And how about this from **World Masters Powerlifting champion and Parrillo Performance Press editor, Marty Gallagher:**

"Pavel Tsatsouline has burst onto the American health and fitness scene like a Russian cyclone. He razes the sacred temples of fitness complacency and smugness with his revolutionary concepts and ideas. If you want a new and innovative approach to the age old dilemma of physical transformation, you've struck the mother-lode."

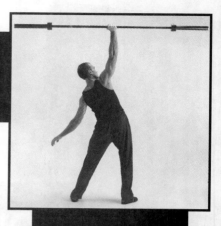

- How to get super strong without training to muscle failure or exhaustion
- How to hack into your 'muscle software' and magnify your power and muscle definition
- How to get super strong <u>without putting on an ounce of weight</u>
- Or how to build massive muscles with a classified Soviet Special Forces workout
- Why high rep training to the 'burn' is like a form of rigor mortis— and what it really takes to develop spectacular muscle tone
- How to mold your whole body into an off-planet rock with only two exercises
- How to increase your bench press by ten pounds overnight
- How to get a tremendous workout on the road without any equipment
- How to design a world class body in your basement—with $150 worth of basic weights and in twenty minutes a day
- How futuristic techniques can squeeze more horsepower out of your body-engine
- How to maximize muscular tension for traffic-stopping muscular definition
- How to minimize fatigue and get the most out of your strength training
- How to ensure high energy after your workout
- How to get stronger and harder without getting bigger
- Why it's safer to use free weights than machines
- How to achieve massive muscles <u>and</u> awesome strength—if that's what you want
- What, how and when to eat for maximum gains
- How to master the magic of effective exercise variation
- The ultimate formula for strength
- How to gain beyond your wildest dreams—with less chance of injury
- A high intensity, immediate gratification technique for massive strength gains
- The eight most effective breathing habits for lifting weights
- The secret that separates elite athletes from 'also-rans'
- How to become super strong and live to tell about it

"You are not training if you are not training with Pavel!"

—Dr. Fred Clary, National Powerlifting Champion and World Record Holder.

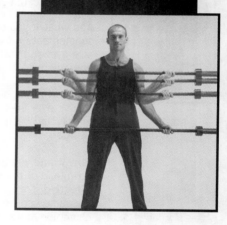

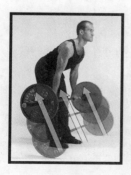

Russians have always made do with simple solutions without compromising the results. NASA aerospace types say that while America sends men to the moon in a Cadillac, Russia manages to launch them into space in a tin can. Enter the tin can approach to designing a world class body—in your basement with $150 worth of equipment. After all, US gyms are stuffed with hi-tech gear, yet it is the Russians with their metal junkyard training facilities who have dominated the Olympics for decades.

Yes, I Want My Fried Abs NOW!— I'm Done Wasting My Time with Slow Burns and Half-Baked Results

As a former Soviet Union Special Forces conditioning coach, Pavel Tsatsouline already knew a thing or two about how to create bullet-stopping abs. Since then, he has combed the world to pry out this select group of primevally powerful ab exercises—guaranteed to yield the fastest, most effective results known to man. According to Pavel, "Crunches belong on the junk pile of history, next to Communism. 'Feeling the burn' with high reps is a waste of time!" Save yourself countless hours of unrewarding, if not useless—if not damaging—toil. Get with the program. Make fast gains and achieve blistering, rock-hard abs now.

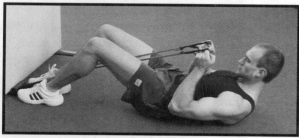

Fry your abs without the spine-wrecking, neck-jerking stress of traditional crunches—using this radical situp designed by the world's leading back and muscle function expert, Professor Janda, from Czechoslovakia.

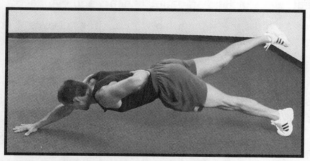

When it came to wanting titanium abs yesterday, the Soviet Special Forces didn't believe in delayed gratification. Pavel gave them what they wanted. If you want abs that'll put you in the world's top 1 percent, this cruel and unusual drill does the trick.

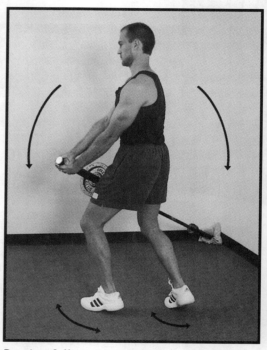

Russian full contact fighters used this drill to pound their opponents with organ-rupturing power, while turning their own midsections into concrete.

1-800-899-5111
24 HOURS A DAY
FAX YOUR ORDER (970) 872-3862

No one—but no one—has ever matched Bruce Lee's ripped-beyond-belief abs. What was his favorite exercise? Here it is. Now you can rip your own abs to eye-popping shreds and reclassify yourself as superhuman.

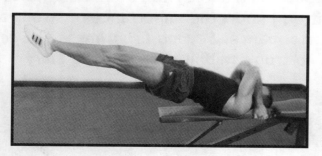

"Are Your Abs Bullet-Proof?"

Introducing the Ab Pavelizer— the fastest, safest way to a ripped powerhouse of six-pack muscle

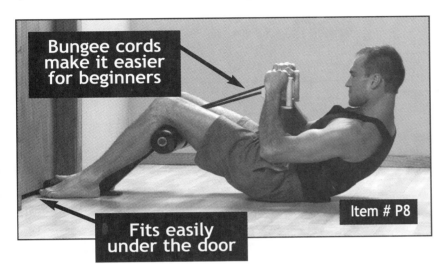

Bungee cords make it easier for beginners

Fits easily under the door

Item # P8

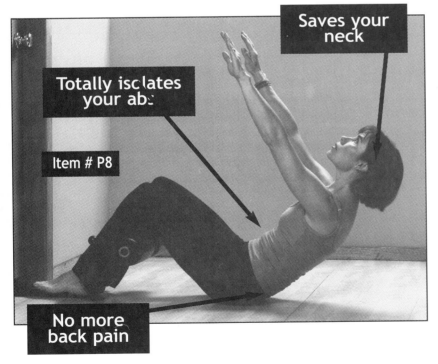

Saves your neck

Totally isolates your abs

Item # P8

No more back pain

In his groundbreaking book *Beyond Crunches: Hard Science. Hard Abs.*—and in the new companion video—Russian Special Forces conditioning coach **Pavel Tsatsouline** reveals the Janda situp, the world's safest and most effective situp. Leading back and muscle function expert, Professor Janda discovered the secret to true ab strength—how to scientifically isolate the abs by "taking out" the hip flexors.

The result: an awesome exercise that scorches the abs, while avoiding the spine-wrecking, neck-jerking antics of traditional (read: outmoded) situps.

Until now, the Janda situp required a partner, for correct form. But with the introduction of the **Ab Pavelizer,** you can quickly develop world-class abs without having to rely on a friend. Now it's strictly between you and your abs. In just a few minutes a day, you can own the world—**ABSOLUTELY.**

To Take Possession of Your New Abs Call This Number Today: 1-800-899-5111

"It Has Never Been So Easy to Have UNGODLY ABS"

This absolute ab machine is available in two versions:

The Ab Pavelizer—Stand Alone

The stand alone version allows you to attach a weight (you won't need more than 50 lbs.) to anchor the machine while you do your partner-free Janda sit up. You will not be able to fit this version under a door.

Item # P8A $159.95 plus $14.00 SH.

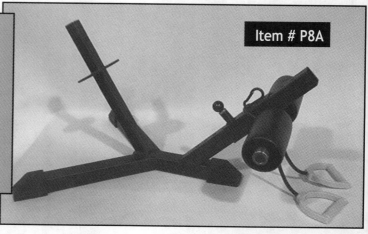

Item # P8A

The Ab Pavelizer

Easily fits under a door for a partner-free Janda sit up.

Item # P8 $119.95 plus $12.00 SH.

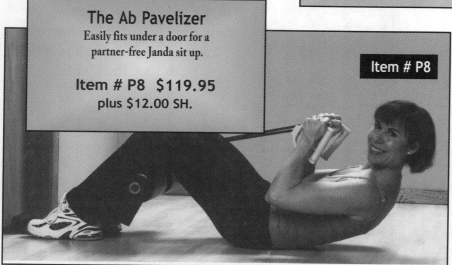

Item # P8

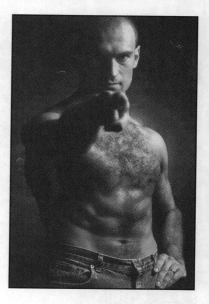

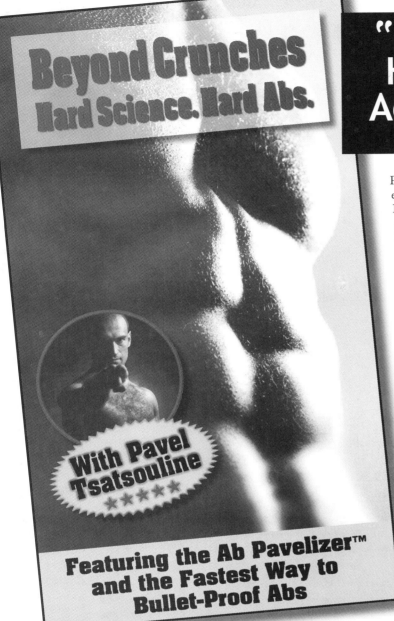

"An Iron Curtain Has Descended Across Your Abs"

Possess a maximum impact training tool for the world's most effective abs, no question.

Includes detailed follow-along instructions on how to perform most of the exercises described in the companion book, *Beyond Crunches*. Demonstrates advanced techniques for optimizing results with the Ab Pavelizer.

As a former Soviet Union Special Forces conditioning coach, **Pavel Tsatsouline** already knew a thing or two about how to create bullet-stopping abs. Since then, he has combed the world to pry out this select group of primevally powerful ab exercises—guaranteed to yield the fastest, most effective results known to man.

- **Fry your abs without the spine-wrecking, neck-jerking stress of traditional crunches.**
- No one—but no one—has ever matched Bruce Lee's ripped-beyond-belief abs. What was his favorite exercise? Here it is. Now you can rip your own abs to eye-popping shreds and reclassify yourself as superhuman.
- Russian fighters used this drill, *The Full-Contact Twist*, to increase their striking power and toughen their midsections against blows. An awesome exercise for iron-clad obliques.
- Rapidly download extreme intensity into your situps—with explosive breathing secrets from Asian martial arts.
- Employ a little-known secret from East German research to radically strengthen your situp.
- Do the right thing with "the evil wheel", hit the afterburners and rocket from half-baked to fully-fried abs.
- "Mercy Me!" your obliques will scream when you torture them with the *Saxon Side Bend*.

• How and why to <u>never, never</u> be nice to your abs—and why they'll love you for it.

• A complete workout plan for optimizing your results from the Janda situp and other techniques.

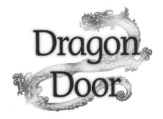

Complete and mail with full payment to:
Dragon Door Publications, P.O. Box 4381, St. Paul, MN 55104

✍ Please print
SOLD TO: *(Street address for delivery)* **A**

Name_____

Street_____

City _____-_____

State _____ Zip _____

Day phone*_____

* Important for clarifying questions on orders

✍ Please print
SHIP TO: *(Street address for delivery)* **A**

Name_____

Street_____

City _____-_____

State _____ Zip _____

Day phone*_____

* Important for clarifying questions on orders

Item #	Qty.	Item Description	Item Price	A or B	Total
P8		Ab Pavelizer	$119.95		
P8A		Ab Pavelizer Stand Alone	$159.95		
V90		Beyond Crunches Video	$29.95		
V51		Beyond Stretching Video	$29.95		
B08		Beyond Crunches Book	$34.95		
B09		Beyond Stretching Book	$34.95		
B10		Power To The People!	$34.95		

HANDLING AND SHIPPING CHARGES
Total Amount of Order Add:

	$00.00 to $24.99	add $5.00	Canada &
	$25.00 to $39.99	add $6.00	Mexico add
	$40.00 to $59.99	add $7.00	$4.00.
NO	$60.00 to $99.99	add $10.00	All other
COD's	$100.00 to $129.99	add $12.00	countries
	$130.00 to $169.99	add $14.00	triple
	$170.00 to $199.99	add $16.00	U.S. charges.
	$200.00 to $299.99	add $18.00	
	$300.00 and up	add $20.00	

Total of Goods	
Shipping Charges	
Rush Charges	
MN residents add 7.0 % sales tax	
Total Enclosed	

Method of Payment ☐ Check ☐ M.O. ☐ Mastercard ☐ Visa ☐ Discover ☐ Diner's Club ☐ Amex

Account No. *(Please indicate all the numbers on your credit card)*   EXPIRATION DATE

☐☐☐☐ ☐☐☐☐ ☐☐☐☐ ☐☐☐☐   ☐☐/☐☐

Day Phone (___) _____

SIGNATURE _____ DATE _____

NOTE: If you wish us to ship by UPS, we must have your street address. Foreign orders are sent by Air Printed Matter. Credit card or International M.O. only.

For rush processing of your order, add an additional $5.00 per address.
Available on money order & charge card orders only.

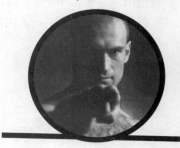

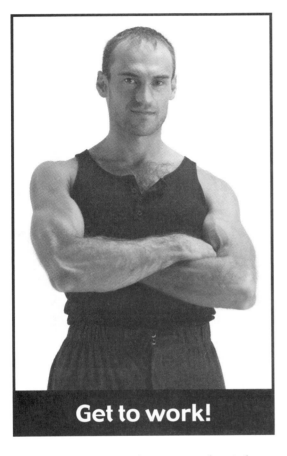

Get to work!

About the Author
Pavel Tsatsouline
Master of Sports

Pavel Tsatsouline, Master of Sports, is a former physical training instructor for Spetsnaz, the Soviet Special Forces, an articulate speaker, and an iconoclastic authority on flexibility and strength training. Pavel was nationally ranked in the Russian ethnic strength sport of kettle-bell lifting and holds a Soviet Physical Culture Institute degree in physiology and coaching. Tsatsouline has authored three books, *Beyond Stretching*, *Beyond Crunches*, and *Power to the People!*

'The Evil Russian' also spreads Communist sports and fitness training propaganda through tailored workshops in a variety of athletic, corporate, and public settings. For seminar availability please e-mail to Pavelizer@aol.com or write to:

ADVANCED FITNESS SOLUTIONS, Inc.
P.O. Box 65472
St. Paul, MN 55165
or
pavelizer@aol.com

NOTES

NOTES

NOTES

NOTES

NOTES

NOTES

NOTES